Gretchen W. TenBrook

Broken Bodies, Healing Hearts
Reflections of a Hospital Chaplain

Pre-publication
REVIEWS,
COMMENTARIES,
EVALUATIONS . . .

"**B**roken bodies . . . bodies torn apart by disease; bodies torn apart by aging; bodies torn apart by trauma; bodies torn apart by life in the workplace; bodies torn apart by death.

These have always been the stories in health care, but now the stories are muffled by managed care, pressures of time, calculations of budget, and not enough time in the day. Time vs. stories. Another brokenness.

This very special book reminds all of us of the stories, and especially of the important work that chaplains are still called to do . . . to identify, hear, and affirm stories and people. It is the pathway to the *healing heart.*"

Rev. Dr. Richard B. Gilbert
Executive Director,
The World Pastoral Care Center,
Valparaiso, IN

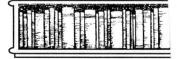

D1307401

"What is it like in a modern urban medical center? We usually imagine Medivac helicopters, high-tech equipment, and the intercom paging busy doctors in long white lab coats. But what is it like for a patient who is waiting for a kidney or a heart, or a man who has lost part of his face to surgery, or a mother whose child is dying of leukemia? Gretchen TenBrook's brief reminiscences will tell you. As a chaplain she has been at their bedside, in the darkness of their rooms and hearts.

And what is it like for the chaplain to stand in the midst of pain, to sit with the suffering, to pray with those grieving the often senseless and irretrievable loss of a loved one? Gretchen shares her deep emotional journey and her personal spiritual struggles in a world where strength and weakness, courage and fear, life and death meet head on.

But these are not vignettes of hopelessness and despair. Over and over we are reminded of the light that shines in the darkness, the strength that comes unannounced and unpredictable, and the love that surrounds the patients, their families, and the chaplain herself. As you read these brief stories of pastoral caring you will feel profoundly inspired by how hearts can heal when bodies are broken."

Rev. P. Barrett Rudd, DMin
Supervisor,
Association for Clinical
Pastoral Education,
Lutherville, MD

"All those visiting 'broken bodies' will find Gretchen TenBrook's writing a source of learning and inspiration. Her self-disclosing and well-expressed style is not only about seeking, but about being found . . . . 'Even though I witness daily God's transforming power in the lives of others, somehow I am still always surprised when it befalls me.' In her goal 'to create an open space for God to live within me' . . . she reveals the human side of courage, the spiritual side of grace."

Ronald P. Dieter, DMin
Licensed Pastoral Psychotherapist,
American Baptist Clergy,
Concord, NH

Broken Bodies, Healing Hearts

*Reflections
of a Hospital Chaplain*

THE HAWORTH PASTORAL PRESS
Religion and Mental Health
Harold G. Koenig, MD
Senior Editor

New, Recent, and Forthcoming Titles:

A Gospel for the Mature Years: Finding Fulfillment by Knowing and Using Your Gifts by Harold Koenig, Tracy Lamar, and Betty Lamar

Is Religion Good for Your Health? The Effects of Religion on Physical and Mental Health by Harold Koenig

Adventures in Senior Living: Learning How to Make Retirement Meaningful and Enjoyable by J. Lawrence Driskill

Dying, Grieving, Faith, and Family: A Pastoral Care Approach by George W. Bowman

The Pastoral Care of Depression: A Guidebook by Binford W. Gilbert

Understanding Clergy Misconduct in Religious Systems: Scapegoating, Family Secrets, and the Abuse of Power by Candace R. Benyei

What the Dying Teach Us: Lessons on Living by Samuel Lee Oliver

The Pastor's Family: The Challenges of Family Life and Pastoral Responsibilities by Daniel L. Langford

Somebody's Knocking at Your Door: AIDS and the African-American Church by Ronald Jeffrey Weatherford and Carole Boston Weatherford

Grief Education for Caregivers of the Elderly by Junietta Baker McCall

The Obsessive-Compulsive Disorder: Pastoral Care for the Road to Change by Robert M. Collie

The Pastoral Care of Children by David H. Grossoehme

Ways of the Desert: Becoming Holy Through Difficult Times by William F. Kraft

Caring for a Loved One with Alzheimer's Disease: A Christian Perspective by Elizabeth T. Hall

"Martha, Martha": How Christians Worry by Elaine Leong Eng

Spiritual Care for Children Living in Specialized Settings: Breathing Underwater by Michael F. Friesen

Broken Bodies, Healing Hearts: Reflections of a Hospital Chaplain by Gretchen W. TenBrook

Shared Grace: Therapists and Clergy Working Together by Marion Bilich, Susan Bonfiglio, and Steven Carlson

The Pastor's Guide to Psychiatric Disorders and Mental Health Resources by W. Brad Johnson and William L. Johnson

Broken Bodies, Healing Hearts
Reflections of a Hospital Chaplain

Gretchen W. TenBrook

The Haworth Pastoral Press
An Imprint of The Haworth Press, Inc.
New York • London • Oxford

Published by

The Haworth Pastoral Press, an imprint of The Haworth Press, Inc., 10 Alice Street, Binghamton, NY 13904-1580

Cover design by Jennifer M. Gaska.

Library of Congress Cataloging-in-Publication Data

TenBrook, Gretchen W.
    Broken bodies, healing hearts : reflections of a hospital chaplain / Gretchen W. TenBrook.
        p.   cm.
    ISBN 0-7890-0851-3 (hc. : alk. paper)—ISBN 0-7890-0852-1 (pbk. : alk. paper)
    1. Spiritual life—Christianity. 2. Christian life. I. Title.

BV4501.2 .T39 2000
248.8'92—dc21
                                                                    99-055440

CONTENTS

Foreword

Gretchen TenBrook is a sensitive, caring, and, above all, very spiritual person who with her unique artistry paints for us the inner world of the hospital chaplain-patient relationship. It is a world of sadness and tragedy, but paradoxically punctuated with beauty, joy, and hope. Tenderly tiptoeing into the patients' lives, with their permission, Chaplain TenBrook allows them to explore their pathos, unbelief, and anger. The stories are powerful and pierce the soul. Gracing each and every patient with dignity, Gretchen presents those to whom she ministers as professors or experts of their own experiences. As a result, they teach us about tolerance, forebearance, what it means to wait . . . about life in general.

Gretchen shows us that hospitals and churches are similar. She states, "We come to both institutions with open wounds, some visible and some not, desperately seeking the remedies buried somewhere in the shambles of our lives." Central to Gretchen's philosophy of care is the sacrament of the Eucharist, for in the broken and bleeding body of Christ, she touches the wounds of the patients as well as her own. The book ends with a triumph of joy as a very ill lady wearing pink silk pajamas transcends her pain and challenges Chaplain Gretchen to change the drabness of her dress, of her very approach to life. In the true essence of ministry, Gretchen receives this woman's advice graciously and the next day arrives on the ward dressed in brilliant colors, only to find an empty hospital room awaiting her. Despite this woman's tragic death, Gretchen finds through a time of bittersweet reflection how her vibrant spirit lives on.

The book is compassionate, joyous, and hopeful. But most of all, it is a beautiful treasury of the soul's journey to God. Read it and be challenged to face the journey of your own soul.

David F. Allen, MD, MPH
Arlington, Virginia
Author of *In Search of the Heart* (1993)
and *Shattering the Gods Within* (1994)

ABOUT THE AUTHOR

Gretchen W. TenBrook is a former Adjunct Chaplain in the Department of Pastoral Care at The Johns Hopkins Hospital in Baltimore, Maryland. She is an affiliate of the Association of Professional Chaplains and has served in pastoral care ministry at several Baltimore hospitals. She is currently working on another book about the call to freedom and surrender in the spiritual life.

Preface

I did not write this book. Rather, through the Spirit's leading, it wrote itself. In this way, it has not been as much an achievement or act of the will as it has been a work of obedience and surrender.

Writing has always been a trustworthy place of fruitful exploration for me. In it, I find a refuge for reflection, and through it, I find a path to the voice of God inside of me. I do not come up with answers as much as I do the genuine questions that lie behind them. And any clarity that befalls me is subject to further refinement, inviting me to continue to seek the ever-new shades of God's eternal light. On the surface, such a pursuit may seem pointless. However, I have found just the opposite to be true, for to participate in divine activity is to willingly go and not to incessantly arrive.

Each essay in this book found its birthplace in the unique story of a person that stirred up a passion within me to wrestle with it in words. As a chaplain in a large academic inner-city hospital, I come into contact with a multitude of people facing a multitude of events amid a multitude of thoughts and emotions. Together, they paint an awesome collage of what it means to be human, *and* what it means to be of divine descent. Needless to say, I find myself constantly walking on fertile ground for spiritual growth, not only for the patients to whom I minister, but also for me.

In my book, I seek to express my heart's true desires, desires that have been made real to me through my visits with patients. In offering a safe place for others simply to be, I have found that God opens my eyes to new horizons of learning about myself, others, and the world in which we live. It is my hope that my book will encourage you to do the same—to look for God's immanent presence in both the momentous and the everyday experiences of life.

I recently wrote the poem "My Heart's Desire." It is a collection of longings that, through the process of writing this book, I have sensed welling up in the very hidden place where only God can touch me. Each desire that has risen to the surface I consider a gift from God, revealed to me through all those who have been courageous enough to let His light shine from their broken hearts: patients and colleagues, friends, family, and strangers alike. May this book invite you, also, to receive the desires of your hearts, desires that find their fulfillment in the very hands of the One who has made them.

MY HEART'S DESIRE

To create an open space for God to live within me.

To empty myself of myself so that He can fill me up.

To wait for my Provider in hopeful expectation.

To be willing to be silent that I may truly hear His still small voice inside me.

To be open to the change of the One who never changes.

To let my false answers become true questions.

To know God's peace in my uncertainty.

To surrender my will for His.

To abandon the shelter of my own making to find myself already inside the mighty house of God.

To offer others a safe place where they are free to come, free to go, and free to be who God made them to be.

To allow others to be true guests in the home of my heart rather than possessions or projects.

To be truly present with others, not subscribing to the illusion that I can fulfill them or they me.

To keep those around me in God's care rather than subject them to my own manipulations.

To move forward with my fellow sojourners rather than to remain in a closed huddle with them.

To find my deepest desires met in God's promises.

To look beyond my idols to the true Source of all my needs.

To find that the Love I so desperately seek is already waiting to be received in my heart.

To know God's presence deeply, even in light of His absence.
To know that the God I can't touch is already touching me.
To know that He who has already come will come again.

To live my humanness to the fullest, just as Jesus did.
To find rest in places of fear, loneliness, and anger, knowing
    that God's healing lies beneath the surface of their roots.
To live the cross that I may live the resurrection.
To see my own illusions shattered by the truth of God's perfect
    provision.
To experience God's kingdom as superior to my own worldly
    longings.

Oh, Lord, You who placed these desires in my heart,
Give me Your courage and Your strength;
For my heart's desire is also my greatest fear.
May I find that there is no fear in Your perfect love.

Gretchen W. TenBrook

Acknowledgments

I would like to express my heartfelt gratitude to all those who have blessed me with the gift of themselves: patients, colleagues, mentors, family, friends, and strangers alike. Some of these people know who they are: may you take joy in the fact that God has touched me in a mighty way through you. Others are not aware of the glimpses of divine love that they have participated in shining my way: may they continue to be beautiful and know their own beauty in doing so. Still others I am not yet aware of myself: may God enable me to see His wonderful ways in all people upon whom I set my eyes.

Specifically, I would like to thank my dear and loving husband, John, for always answering "yes" to the question I've asked hundreds of times: "Will you read this?" I am grateful for his Spirit-led insight, and for his patience amid my sometimes willful and stubborn attitude. I am also thankful for his helping me with my "was's" and "were's" and "lays" and "lies." Sorry, Love, but I fear I will never get those straight!

I would also like to express my thanks to all of my Clinical Pastoral Education (CPE) supervisors and fellow students. Your generous participation in my learning and willingness to tackle tough questions with me has been invaluable! The CPE process has been essential to my growth as a chaplain, and as a person in general.

—1—

And a Child Shall Lead Them

The Meyer family had traveled all the way from Texas, only to be told that nothing could be done for their three-year-old son, Jimmy. Nothing, nothing at all. The child had an inoperable brain tumor that had not responded to multiple trials of chemotherapy and radiation. I imagined the growth inside of his head, spreading its toxic tentacles like an octopus seizing a long-awaited meal.

I came upon Jimmy and his mother in the pediatric playroom. As I was making my rounds on the ward, I heard the sound of clattering toys. I peered into the playroom and was immediately taken with a sight that left me temporarily mesmerized. Jimmy was running in circles around the room, dragging a blue plastic wagon filled with blankets and an oversized stuffed bear. The sturdy cart was normally his mode of transportation, faithfully pulled by his mother on the frequent days when he didn't feel so well. It was evident that Jimmy took great pride in doing himself what his mother usually did for him.

Mrs. Meyer sat perched on the windowsill, her tear-stained eyes staring off into the distance. I wondered what she was thinking about: what the doctors had said, what it would be like without her son, how much time the family had left together? In any case, she seemed to be avoiding participating in Jimmy's play, as if it would be too painful to enjoy what would soon be taken from her.

While Mrs. Meyer's thoughts appeared to be traveling into the inevitable future that she dreaded, Jimmy's mind remained focused on the only thing he knew—the moment at hand. "Whew!" he sang gleefully, followed by a giggle, watching the wagon temporarily escape the command of his little hand. Jimmy's ignorance of his terminal illness appeared to be a blessing, his innocent mind not yet subject to the distortions of a world of worries. Unlike his mother, and unlike me, Jimmy seemed to possess an ability to live fully in the joy of the moment. He reminded me of the children who, having witnessed Jesus' healing power, shouted, "Hosanna to the Son of David!" (Matthew 21:14-16).* While the chief priests and teachers worried about the implications of those words, the children simply celebrated them for the sense of exultation they brought to the very moment. Jesus, citing the words of King David, then proclaimed in response what had already been written: "From the lips of children and infants, you have ordained praise" (Matthew 21:16, Psalm 8:2).

As I watched Jimmy carelessly roam the room like any healthy toddler, I wondered how he could be terminally ill. Surely the same question had crossed Mrs. Meyer's mind countless times on the rare days when her little one was blessed with such boundless energy. By the grace of God, Jimmy was not at a point to understand his grave situation, only to simply receive whatever it brought each day and the next. In his simple trust, I saw the kingdom of heaven. In his very being, I was encouraged to grow up in my own faith and become like a child.

While part of me felt a tremendous sense of peace in watching Jimmy, another part of me felt ill. I was angry that the precious little boy that the Meyer family had been granted was likely to be taken away just a few years after his birth. One day soon, Jimmy's head would no longer be able to accommodate the ever-increasing tumor, leaving his life-preserving brain tissue vulnerable prey to the insatiable appetite of the growth. According to the doctors, it was only a matter of time. "Why Jimmy? Why Jimmy?" I raged at God inside my head, recognizing that my anger was probably miniscule compared to that of Mrs. Meyer. But then, in the midst of my frantic questioning, another perspective seemed to settle into my thoughts with the clarity of a flashlight shown into a dark hole. "Why not Jimmy?" I heard. "Why not Jimmy?" Yes, Jimmy was young and cherished, but who was I to say that his life was more valuable than another's? Who was I to decide who could rightly die and who couldn't? To be angry at God was an understandable response, but to try to play God was a waste of time and energy.

---

*All quoted scripture is from *The Holy Bible,* NIV Study Bible, 1985. Grand Rapids, MI: Zondervan Publishing House.

I was suddenly arrested from my sea of thoughts by a loud crash. I immediately looked up to find Jimmy restoring the toppled wagon and picking up Bear, the fuzzy brown stuffed animal that had been thrown out during the collision. He carefully placed Bear back on the blankets and then resumed towing the wagon as if nothing had happened. For Jimmy, the calamity simply seemed like an integral part of his play, just as suffering had most likely always played a regular role in his life.

Aroused from her trance by the discord, Mrs. Meyer looked to me expectantly. I walked into the room and introduced myself, initially greeted by Jimmy. The toddler stopped his play momentarily and stared up at me with a friendly grin. In his glowing face, so full of genuine hope and void of harmful presuppositions, I felt the warmth of God shine on me with the intensity of a heat lamp. "And whoever welcomes a little child like this in my name welcomes me" I could hear Jesus speaking to my heart (Matthew 18:5).

Jimmy's delightful expression served as a powerful complement to his bald and swollen head, which resembled a giant cantaloupe, big enough to knock the rest of his little body off balance. In his unique appearance, I saw the poles of suffering and joy, of death and new life, converge into a harmonious whole.

Mrs. Meyer responded nervously to my introduction. "Hi," she said in a shaky voice, looking down at the floor as if to hide her grief-stricken face. Interestingly, Jimmy appeared not to be affected by his mother's display of emotion, at least on a conscious level. Perhaps he had grown accustomed to tears now, realizing that they were simply a part of life.

"We better go meet Daddy in the cafeteria," Mrs. Meyer suddenly blurted, gathering her belongings. It was clear to me that she didn't want to talk or even spend time with me. Perhaps she saw me as additional confirmation of her son's dreary fate, another messenger of the bad news. I flexed accordingly with her plans, knowing that only she could dictate the process of her own grieving.

"Pastoral care services are always available to you if you have any need," I mentioned as she made her way toward the door, lugging several bags in one hand and the wagon handle in the other. "Thank you," she responded in a brief yet sincere tone. Jimmy and Bear sat contentedly in the wagon, the little boy waving to me as they rounded the corner into the hallway.

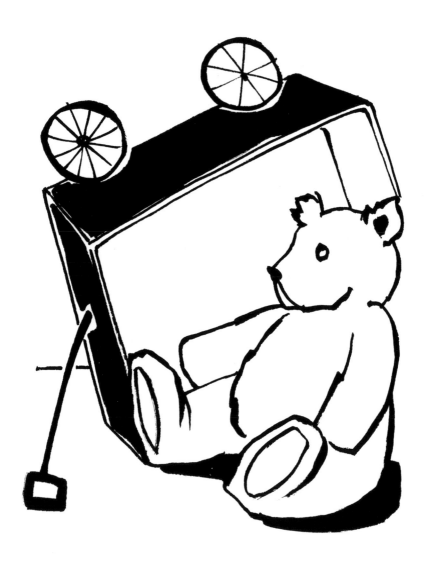

—2—

Beyond Pity

A gentle knock sounded on the conference room door. I collapsed into the back of my chair and let out a deep sigh of frustration, for just when I had managed to find some free time for my writing, I was immediately interrupted. But then through the grace of God, I remembered that my time is not my own, but rather God's to be used for His own purposes. "So what will you have for me now, Lord?" I thought to myself as I got up to answer the door.

A short and plump middle-aged woman appeared before me, looking up at me with a heaviness that spoke of shame and despair. Her eyes were partly covered by a black hat that sealed her head like a pen cap. I wondered if her hat gave her the security that her tattered heart could not. She was dressed in a ratty Orioles sweatshirt and untied tennis shoes, both worn from what I imagined were endless days of wandering the city streets for something that couldn't be found there. I sensed that her ragged appearance was a reflection of the brokenness she felt inside. Perhaps she was on the verge of realizing that she could no longer take care of herself. Little did she know she was headed in the right direction.

"Hi. My name's Linda," she muttered. "I just really need to talk to someone here." She looked up at me in a plea for help.

"Come on in, Linda," I replied, wanting to provide a safe place of hospitality for her. She quickly made her way to the nearest chair, eyeing the challah rolls on the table reserved for that day's Sabbath service. In a strange way, I wanted to offer her one, knowing that it was indeed bread for the needy. Instead, however, I decided that we were free to seek God's nourishment in its countless other forms.

"I was thinking we could pray and then maybe . . . maybe go to the cafeteria," she quickly yet hesitantly petitioned, anxiously scanning the room around us. "I mean, I don't really have any money, but maybe you could get me just a little something."

"Okay," I responded with a gentle smile and a nod, wanting to offer her a bit of control amid her chaos. At the same time, however, I wondered if my willingness to accommodate her was simply serving as a deposit into a bankrupt account of manipulation. Just how many people had she approached with such pleas, thinking that, like shots of cocaine, their temporary provisions would solve all of her problems? Disappointed over and over again, she would lock herself into a circle of empty promises. Despite my uncertainty, I decided to give Linda the benefit of the doubt, remembering that no matter where she was on her journey toward God, she still needed the light of His grace to lead her way.

As I watched Linda squirming in the seat next to me, I thought of Jean Valjean, the released prisoner in Victor Hugo's *Les Misérables*. Marked as a convict forever, he finally found shelter in the home of a compassionate bishop. In the middle of the night, he robbed the kind man of his silver and fled just before daybreak. The police eventually caught Jean and brought him back to the bishop. In his mercy, the bishop simply gazed into the eyes of his offender and cheerfully asked him why he had forgotten to take the candlesticks, as well. The policemen released him from his shackles, and Jean's life was forever changed through the power of grace. I only hoped that one day Linda, too, would receive the grace that would be forever extended her way.

It didn't take long for Linda to unload her story. Tragedy after tragedy gushed from her lips, as if our meeting were the only context in which they could be spewed forth. "Well, my boyfriend of twenty-three years, he gone with some other woman. And my children, I got three, but they don't love me anymore. One got taken away, adopted. One fell out of a window. The other, I just never see him. I'm just so pitiful." She laid her load of troubles on the table. before us and then paused, as if she expected me to pick them up and repackage them into a tidy arrangement that she could store away forever. Little did she know that the peace she sought was in the midst of her pain, that the answers she looked for were buried amid the complexity of her questions.

"I was in here for two weeks for depression, you know, but now I'm out and I don't know what to do," she continued, seemingly trying to push herself further into the illusion that someone else had all of the answers to her questions and solutions to her problems. "I'm just so pitiful, so pitiful," she continued, caught in the rut of a destructive self-image. It occurred to me that the evil one had her right where he wanted her.

Hoping to shatter her notions in order to give way to Truth, I simply acknowledged her pain and asked her what she would like to include in prayer. She looked at me, as if somewhat confused by my question. "Aren't you supposed to know that?" I could hear her saying to herself. Yes, I could speculate, but such prayers usually end up as attempts to fill my own needs rather than those of the patient.

After a brief prayer "for everything," we made our way to the cafeteria. Linda hastily picked out a soda and a cream cheese pastry. Again, she was seeking nourishment from sources that tasted good for the moment, but had no lasting value. I wanted to say, "How about a bagel and some orange juice instead?" but then I realized that I could only provide a place for her to choose, not make the choices for her.

Linda sat down at the nearest table, the food seemingly more important than the company during the meal. I watched her wolf down her pastry in a matter of seconds, and then commented, "Linda, you are *really* hungry." She just nodded, her mouth too full for words. Little did she know that I was speaking of a different hunger, a far more intense hunger that only manifested itself in pastries, people, things, places, everything—everything except God. Unfortunately, I sensed that Linda was too frantically full of her own temporary solutions to allow God's lasting solution to fill her.

"Do you have any spare change?" she asked after her last bite of pastry, seeming to already need another fix. I mindlessly reached into my purse and pulled out a dollar. As I handed it to her, I heard the Voice inside me say, "That's not what she needs!" But the moment had passed and it was too late. I, too, was weak, and in my ignorance I sought comfort in the illusion that I could be her savior. Linda and I were more alike than I wished to believe. I only hoped that she, too, would be set free with the knowledge that only God holds the keys to the desires of our hearts.

As we made our way to the cafeteria exit, Linda seemed rushed and anxious. I wondered just where she was planning to go next. Moreover, I wondered just how long she would choose to forfeit the gift of God's mighty home for her own useless shelters.

"I wish God listened to my prayers. I don't think He listens to prayers from people like me. I bet he listens to you, though. I'm just so pitiful," she muttered with each hasty step.

I stopped in my tracks and leaned up against the side of the hallway, deciding that I was not going to reinforce the harness of pity in which she was imprisoning herself. I, too, had been down that road before, presenting myself to others as helpless in an attempt to get their reassurance, in an attempt to get them to do for me what I needed to do for myself. How challenging and humbling, yet freeing and renewing it was to realize that if I was willing to see myself as God's beloved, then my self-hatred would be transformed into a newfound humility.

"So you think you're pitiful," I reflected.

She nodded and then shook her head in shame.

"And?" I queried, inviting her to remove the blinders she had tied in knots around her head. Linda just looked at me in a blank stare. Apparently, she didn't get it.

"What do you mean, 'And?'" she asked, wrinkling her nose as if my question stunk. I hoped that one day she would smell the sweet essence of God's grace in the memory of my words. I asked her what she thought I meant, and she continued to look confused.

"Well, the God I know came for the sick, not the well," I bluntly offered to Linda. "And I don't think I've ever met a single person who doesn't suffer from some sort of illness. So when I say 'And?' I'm asking you what you will choose to do with your situation." I looked directly into her eyes, hoping to convey that the decision was hers to make. Linda then looked down at the floor, as if she were attempting to skirt the pivotal question.

"Can I give you some food for thought?" I queried, sensing a piece of scripture descending into my mind. She nodded, as much to accept the offer as to escape the discomfort of the moment. In our refuge lane amid the traffic of the hallway, I pulled out a copy of the

Gideon's New Testament from my bag and opened it to the book of Hebrews.

" 'For we do not have a high priest who is unable to sympathize with our weaknesses,' " I began reading, " 'but we have one who has been tempted in every way, just as we are—yet was without sin. Let us then approach the throne of grace with confidence, so that we may receive mercy and find grace to help us in our time of need' " (Hebrews 4:15-16).

"Hmm," Linda muttered. I wasn't sure whether her response indicated that she was reflecting on the scripture or just attempting to make it look that way. In any case, God's word had been offered, and I trusted that Linda would receive it or not receive it in her own time.

"Here, you can have this," I said, handing to her the *Gideon's New Testament*. Finally, I sensed I was giving to her a tangible item that she *did* need. She took the little book and whispered a thank-you under her breath. She looked up at me in a stoic gaze, appearing to be lost in another world, in a place she had never been before. I caressed her shoulder, smiled gently, and said good-bye, sensing that she was exactly where she needed to be.

—3—

Redeemed by Grace

Mr. Nelson was a picture of grace. His story was one of those rare ones that bring tears to the eyes, chills to the spine, and warmth to the heart. Hearing it was like receiving a gift from heaven—a package wrapped by the hands of God.

I hadn't expected to hear such a beautiful testimony from the lips of this weary man who was recovering from his second heart attack at the relatively young age of forty-nine. With tiny beads of sweat lacing his chin and greasy unkempt locks draping his forehead, he looked as if he had been caught in a hurricane. In a sense, he had. Yet as Mr. Nelson began to share his life with me, the sense of peace with which he spoke seemed to compel the intensity of his ailing condition to fade into the background. Yes, he was sick, but I was to learn that he was also alive and well.

"It was late on a Sunday night, and I was working with several other guys," he began as I settled into the bedside chair. He paused briefly to mention how he'd always felt guilty about working on Sundays instead of going to church. His side comment sounded sincere, yet I wondered if it would have gone unmentioned with another audience.

"We were trying to work on this big expensive piece of machinery that the company had," he continued, "but the other guys—they all fell asleep on the job. It was just me; I was all alone. And I was mad, so mad that I cussed them out! I was steaming. . . . I got mad a lot those days . . ."

Mr. Nelson stared off into the distance and his eyes became glassy, as if reflecting upon painful memories. The burly man had always had trouble controlling the violent behavior that tended to erupt from his anger. He had told me earlier in our visit how it used to dominate his entire life. "I would pick a fight at anything," he had said, shaking his head in disbelief. "So bad I could feel my heart skipping beats."

Mr. Nelson abruptly jerked his head and blinked his eyes repeatedly, as if freeing himself from a prison of the past. He shifted his attention back to me and the story at hand.

"I didn't feel well all of the sudden, and the next thing I knew, I was lying on the floor, breathing hard, my chest pumping up and down . . . just like my father's did when he died."

Just like his father—someone with whom I suspected Mr. Nelson never shared a close bond. Mr. Nelson had spoken of his father earlier during our visit with an odd distance, as if he had never really known him. I wondered what memories and feelings lurked behind his brief words of identification with his father.

"I remember thinking to myself as I was lying there on the floor," Mr. Nelson continued, " 'Well, my life's been hard, so I'll just die now' and that that's all there was to it." Mr. Nelson shrugged his shoulders in resignation as he relived the hopelessness of that moment.

Mr. Nelson *had* had a hard life. Happy times seemed to be limited to his childhood in the care of his mother. He spoke fondly of her. "She always did her best to raise me in a good Christian home," he had said, shaking his head as if remembering the discipline involved, and laughing as if knowing that it was done in love.

Life seemed to sour as Mr. Nelson grew older. He joined the Navy as a young adult and seemed to feel as though the experience had tarnished him. "They lived differently in the Navy, and I just sort of fell into that," he had recalled. I wondered what activities he had been involved in, envisioning a group of drunken sailors throwing beer bottles and women in the dark alleys of a port town. Aware that my mind was headed in the wrong direction, I held my morbid curiosity in check. I knew that what mattered most was not Mr. Nelson's past but, rather, how he felt about it now. And from what I could discern so far, Mr. Nelson seemed to have made peace with his past. He appeared to be able to confront it with an openness and ingenuity that enabled him to move forward to a place of healing and new life.

Continuing his story, Mr. Nelson brought me back to his collapsed position on the factory floor. He explained that after resigning himself to what seemed imminent death, he was overcome by the concept of eternity. "I thought to myself, 'Eternity is forever, and there's no coming back.' I didn't want to leave things the way they were. I thought of my wife and my daughter. I wanted to make things better with them."

Mr. Nelson appeared to be temporarily engulfed in his memories, lying still and silent, as I sat conscientiously at his bedside. I felt like a child waiting to hear the exciting conclusion of an age-old legend passed down through her ancestors.

Mr. Nelson surfaced from his trancelike state and resumed. "I remember looking up from the floor, and seeing all the guys I worked with looking down at me. I was so embarrassed at how I had lashed out at them, at how I'd lashed out at everybody in my life." Mr. Nelson paused, looking down, feeling the disappointment all over again.

Yet Mr. Nelson's disappointment had served to lead him to the door of repentance, and it is there that he then knocked. "Something inside of me was telling me to ask for forgiveness. I thought to myself, 'Okay, I'll just pray silently to God.' But then I remembered the Bible verse my mother had taught me about being accountable before all men, and I knew I had to confess out loud, right then. So I just started praying right there, out loud and all. It's funny: it was all happening so fast, yet I had so many thoughts going through my head."

Just as many other life-changing events I'd heard about, Mr. Nelson's took on a timeless quality. I found myself feeling a bit jealous of his experience, wishing God would speak to me in such a clear fashion. Yet at the same time, I was not the least bit envious of the years of hurt and anger or the eventual heart attack that Mr. Nelson had to experience to get to such a place of divine revelation.

"So God gave me a second chance," he concluded with a chuckle.

"And all you had to do was ask . . ." I noted, reflecting on the grace that had saturated the pivotal moment in his life.

"Yep," Mr. Nelson replied. We looked up at each other and smiled and laughed, consumed by the abundant love of our God whose mercy knows no bounds.

—4—

Divine Identity

Little did Mrs. Jameson know it, but she had come home for the first time without even leaving the hospital. It was a beautiful sight, and I felt honored to be part of the event. Somehow, in the midst of our awkward conversation, she had come to recognize her true identity.

Indeed, a hospital may sound like a strange place to discover that one is made in the image of God. But then again, perhaps not, because it is in such a place where all that boasts no eternal significance is stripped away, leaving only what could be divinely created.

Mrs. Jameson was the type who didn't have much to say. Everything seemed simply humdrum to her, even a potentially fatal episode of fluid overload. "I'm doin' fine . . ." she uttered in monotone voice. I wondered what it would take to awaken her from her slumber. Apparently, a lot. Apparently, Truth and Love. Apparently, God.

"I'm surprised you came in here, to see *me* of all people . . ." Mrs. Jameson sighed. She looked up at me in a lethargic gaze, as if somewhat bewildered and confused.

"Hmm," I responded, wondering what was behind her self-deprecating words. "What makes you say that?"

"Well, I mean . . . there be so many other mo' sicker people here . . . mo' religious ones too. Me . . . I'm just . . . well, I'm just . . . okay." Mrs. Jameson's words slowly dripped from her mouth like ketchup from a glass bottle, hesitantly and void of any purpose.

"You're just . . . *okay?*" I reflected, noticing the insignificance of the word with which she associated herself.

"Yeah . . . " she continued, mumbling under her breath. "I mean . . . I ain't nothin' special or nothin'." The fifty-something woman shrugged her shoulders.

"Well, when I came in here I knew I was about to meet someone God made," I proposed. "I'd say that means you're special, certainly more than just okay." We both just sat there and looked at each other momentarily, pondering the implication of my words. A rich smile slowly took shape on her face, like a morning sun shedding its light on what had previously been enveloped in darkness.

"Really?" she asked me in disbelief. Her animated voice suggested that a new energy had just been breathed into her. As her chin dropped and lips curled, her expression of utter joy reminded me of a giggling baby's, embracing her entire face like a warm blanket. It was as if I had just given to her the best news of her life. Maybe I had.

"You mean . . . you knew that, that I was . . . made by . . . by *God* when you came in here?" She clumsily forced out this idea that I assumed was a new one for her.

"Yep," I responded with a gentle nod. Her need for confirmation surprised me, but then I realized that my mere statement had been a revelation to her, a truth that had never before been met face to face or even contemplated.

Of course, I didn't tell Mrs. Jameson that I see every patient this way: as a unique creation shaped by the hands of God. While I hoped that one day she would realize her membership in this divine community, it seemed enough at the time for her to be embraced by the newfound gift of her own belovedness. Like a caterpillar, she was being nurtured in the safety of her own cocoon. How different I hoped her reality appeared now. Maybe she no longer saw her life as a prison of sickness, but as a refuge for healing; no longer as a stale jar of meaninglessness, but as a sanctuary of purpose; no longer as a battlefield where numbness and apathy were the only protectors from harm, but as a playground where both the thrill of a slide ride and the pain of a skinned knee were welcome to be lived to their fullest.

Mrs. Jameson sank into the pillows behind her, closed her eyes, and smiled. We sat in a silent contemplation that spoke too loudly for words. Part of me longed to push Mrs. Jameson further, to introduce her to the responsibility behind claiming her divine identity, to protect her from the tragedy of distorting what she had just discovered. But deep down I knew that this was God's job, not mine, to be worked out in His own timing.

Yes, Mrs. Jameson had come home for the first time in fifty-plus years of life, stumbling upon the door of love that had long been held ajar awaiting her arrival. However, she had not yet come to understand the nature of the house in which she was to dwell. Where did the roof come from? Which room was hers? With whom did she live? Who cooked the meals and who did the dishes? Such questions were yet to be confronted, let alone answered. But for now, I envisioned Mrs. Jameson simply sitting in front of the fireplace in a rocking chair, enjoying the warmth and comfort of this newfound place of genuine peace. It was time for her to rest and be loved, like a tree whose full, green branches wave freely in the summer breeze. Winter would come in due time, and with it a time to become bare and vulnerable in order to grow anew.

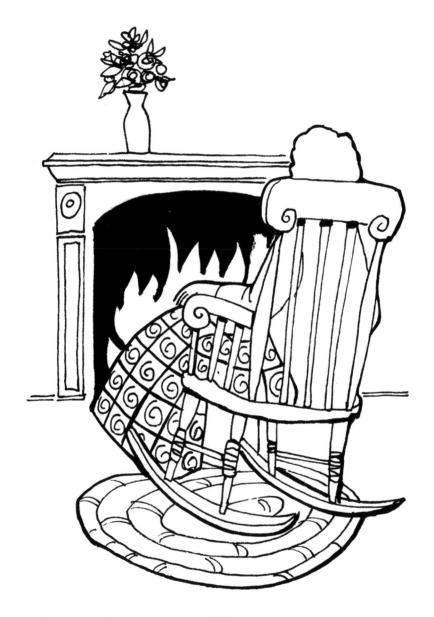

©1999 Michael O'Neill McGrath, OSFS

—5—

Learning to Be

Mr. Stetson couldn't talk, but his physical appearance loudly proclaimed the agony of his condition. A tracheotomy pierced a bloody hole in the fifty-eight-year-old man's throat, through which a ventilator was connected, forcing his chest to rise and fall like an old worn-out machine. His face looked tired and anxious, his eyebrows dripping with sweat and his eyes roaming around the room sporadically. As I stood at his bedside, I wondered what was going through this man's mind. I wondered what it would be like to be alert, awake, and alive, yet unable to breathe. Breathing—something that I have always taken for granted, something I've always considered to be synonymous with life.

"Hello, Mr. Stetson," I said calmly. Suddenly aware that Mr. Stetson would not be able to respond verbally to my greeting, I found myself feeling uncertain of what to say, nervous, uncomfortable, almost nauseous. I wanted to comfort him, not to frustrate him, and I had to decide at that very moment how to go about doing this. I had no choice other than to lean on the grace of God, trusting that He would supply me with the right thoughts, words, and actions.

Eventually, I decided that an introduction was in order, realizing that this suffering man probably had no idea who the young woman in the green floral dress standing ambivalently at his bedside was.

"My name is Gretchen TenBrook, and I'm a chaplain here at the hospital. I'm just coming in to see how you're feeling." I stumbled over my words, wondering how I could best convey a caring presence to Mr. Stetson without making him feel as if he had to perform for me. Somehow, there seemed no easy way, and I sensed that I would have to feel my way, staying true to the present moment and trusting God for the next.

"I know you can't say any . . . that you can't talk," I stuttered, realizing that apparently, neither could I. "But I still wanted you to know that I . . . I am available to support you in any way I can." Mr. Stetson slowly nodded and blinked his eyes in affirmation, as I reflected upon the stale nature of my comment. I wished I had a more genuine way to express what sounded so rehearsed and canned.

Several moments of silence crept by as I stood next to Mr. Stetson, noticing that the room full of high-tech equipment lacked a simple chair. It was still and quiet, with the rude and rhythmic interruption of the wheezing ventilator. It felt cold and hard and inhuman. I wanted to bring some warmth into the room, to bring some hope into the despair, some life into the impending death. How disturbing it was to recognize that there was little I could do for Mr. Stetson. In fact, the only thing I could do was *to be* with him. *To be* with Mr. Stetson: this was the greatest gift I knew I could give to him now, but somehow it didn't seem to be enough.

Part of me wanted to leave, to run out of the room, to call it a day. There were many easier ways I could be spending my time: vegging on the couch in front of Oprah, tackling the pile of laundry in the hamper, baking a batch of my husband's favorite cookies. Such mindless activities suddenly had great appeal as I wallowed in a temporary flush of insecurity. "I feel like an idiot." These words kept flooding my mind like buckets of cold water.

At the same time, I knew that to leave Mr. Stetson at that moment would be a cop-out and a loss, a mere forfeit. Mr. Stetson and I both had something to offer each other, even if not words, and to deny our exchange would be to abandon the work of God's hands. My sense of discomfort with the situation was driving me away, yet my sense of peace called me to stay. The familiar words of one of my mentors that have kept me in countless patients' rooms crossed my mind, yet again. "Remember, Gretchen. You are called to be faithful, not successful."

Suddenly, Mr. Stetson moved his needle-poked hands from beneath the starched sheet, saving me from drowning in my sea of mixed emotions. He slowly brought them together, aligning his fingertips to form a steeple: he wanted to pray. I felt my shoulders drop, my breathing slow, my mind thaw: I was relieved. Mr. Stetson's request for prayer put me at ease and made me feel accepted. Finally, I could *do* something!

I offered my hand to Mr. Stetson and he gently grasped it, closing his eyes to welcome the prayer. The words came, although they were few. There seemed to be only one thing to pray for at that time: peace and comfort for a man whose outlook was matter-of-factly stated by the attending physician as "terminal." Yes, the God I knew was a God of second chances, but also a God of natural endings. Where Mr. Stetson was to be now and to head tomorrow, only God knew. In my heart I prayed that whatever happened, Mr. Stetson would know the presence of the One who gave him life and would one day bring him back home.

The prayer somehow brought our visit to a natural close. I squeezed Mr. Stetson's hand, knowing that there was strength somewhere in his weakness, and headed for the door. As I walked to the nurse's station, I felt full and empty at the same time: full of the rich emotions that his situation had evoked, yet empty of any genuine connection in which I had hoped to partake.

As I plopped into a chair next to a stack of medical records, caught in the typical rush of rounding doctors, frantic nurses, and beeping heart monitors, a wave of disappointment and frustration washed over me, a sort of rude revelation. I wondered if the very thing I had sought while visiting Mr. Stetson was what I had let slip right through my fingers: to trust God in the moment rather than to run to the next, to rest in the place of uncertainty rather than to seek asylum in the place of control, *to be* rather than *to do*. I realized that when Mr. Stetson asked me to pray, I jumped at the opportunity with great relief because it was an escape from the trusting that was so scary, the uncertainty that was so awkward, *the being* that was so foreign to my goal-oriented mind.

"When will I learn just *to be*?" I thought to myself. This struggle was not uncharted territory to me, and deep down, I knew that I would revisit it many times.

—6—

Homecoming

It wasn't the hospital, but in many ways it felt like it: another building full of broken people seeking wholeness and healing in their lives, including me. Yes, hospitals and churches share more in common than one would think. Hopeful yet hurting, we come to both institutions with open wounds, some visible and some not, desperately seeking the remedies buried somewhere in the shambles of our lives.

This is the sense that came over me the moment I walked into church on that cold and clear Sunday morning. Little did I know that the weather was a preview of what was to come: a glimpse of God's clarity, warmth, and light amid the frostbitten landscape of a young woman's life. I noticed her immediately when we walked into the sanctuary and made our way to our seats. She was sitting right behind us, nested on the edge of her chair as if to balance the weight of her body with that of her bursting belly. *Very* pregnant, she looked as though she could go into labor at any moment. She sat snuggled against Penny like a toddler hiding between her mother's legs, as if she feared the rest of the congregation might bite her. Penny was one of the coordinators of Sparrow House, a ministry of the church for pregnant, unwed, teenage mothers who lack family support. Given their proximity, I figured the young woman had sought refuge at this haven where regular prenatal care and emotional support were assured. Once her baby was born, it would be her choice to raise the child, or to put him or her up for adoption.

The young woman was a sharp contrast to the other teens sitting in the back of the church who were dressed in the latest fashions and caught in a series of hushed giggles. Her blonde-dyed hair was pulled tightly up into a bun, exposing her round and rosy cheeks, which resembled mini versions of her stomach. Dressed in leggings and an oversize shirt, and decorated with dangling earrings in multiple orifices, I wondered what she was trying to hide. I sensed that there was something, something else inside of her just waiting to be born.

Carelessly muttering the words of the opening hymn, I found myself unable to concentrate on worship. Instead of the usual frustration I experience with my wandering mind, however, I felt near God, somehow very aware of His immanent presence. I sensed His divine energy from behind me, as if the sun were shining directly on my back. As I glanced over my shoulder, I noticed the young pregnant woman appeared to be in the same place I was: in church yet somewhere very far away in her heart and mind. Perhaps we had more in common than it seemed on the surface. I, married and infertile, she, unmarried and fertile, both looking for some sort of nourishment to satisfy our deep hungers. She, too, lifelessly mouthed the lyrics of the hymn. With eyes red and puffy yet empty, she stared at the back of my chair as if there were something of marked interest there. I sensed that she was desperately searching for something, something that her eyes longed to see but could not as hard as she tried. And from the roots of that search emanated God's warmth, like the radiating beam from a distant lighthouse that enables sailors to chart the night's course.

In some ways, the attraction I felt toward this young woman, whose name I do not know to this day, has confused me. Should I not be finding God's presence in those who appear strong: in the man who prophesies in tongues; in the woman whose breast cancer virtually disappeared from the mammogram; in the sixty-five-year-old who commits his days to volunteer ministry to shut-ins; in the child who can miraculously walk after years of paralysis? Yes, such displays of God's power are indeed inspiring and rare. But ironically, it is often in the company of my fellow broken and vulnerable brothers and sisters that I sense God's presence the most, for we are all wounded in some way by the hurts of life that befall us. Perhaps the reality of the divine is most evident to me in this context because, in my experience, our common suffering has the power to bring us together to a place and time where God's healing may flow freely.

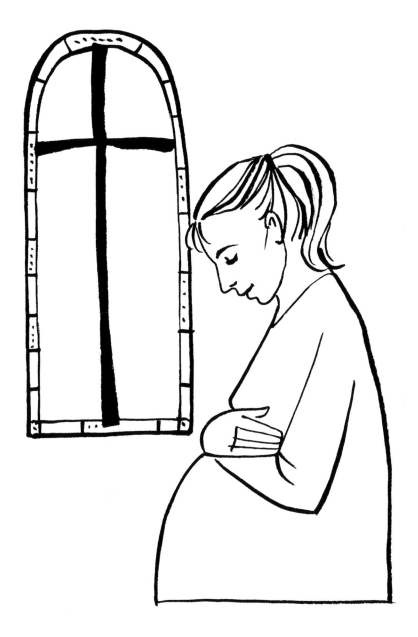

As I gazed at the young woman at church, I didn't see an unwed pregnant teenager, but rather I saw a tender heart longing to be loved, longing to be healed from the wounds of the past. No, I did not know what her situation was, and I didn't need to know. I simply sensed that that day would be a renewing one for her, that she might find light in her darkness and refuge in her desert.

The service proceeded, and I wandered in and out of it, catching an occasional verse in the readings, a random word of hope in the sermon, and a rare catchy chorus in the praise songs. Everything seemed distant and disjointed, except for the certainty of God's presence, whose transcending power made everything okay.

Before I knew it, it was time to approach the altar for communion. My attention sharpened as I looked forward to receiving the sacrament. It serves as a mysterious yet tangible reminder of God's love for me. In the elements I see the body and blood of Christ given up for me; in receiving them into my mouth I hear myself say "yes" to God's grace; in ingesting them into my body I taste my Maker's provision; in reflecting on them in prayer I smell the sweet essence of God's strength and renewal for the days to come.

Apparently, I was not the only one who found communion an exceptionally powerful experience that day. As I returned to my seat, I noticed the young woman making her way toward the altar. No longer frozen in an endless stare, she appeared to be scanning the room vigilantly. She reminded me of a freight train pulling into the station after a long journey. It was time for her cargo to be unloaded, deposited so that she could be refilled with goods that would propel her in the future rather than confine her to the past. Standing in front of the priest, she opened and lifted her shaking hands to receive the host. Her formal yet ragged gesture spoke surrender to me, for as she offered herself to God, He offered Himself to her.

After the Eucharist the young woman approached Jake, one of the Eucharistic ministers who was offering post-communion prayer. She looked like a tearful child about to confess to her mother that she had spilled her milk, longing for a hug but dreading a beating. As Jake placed his hands tenderly on her shoulders and bowed over her, the ravaged teenager's whole body seemed to relax, as if she had removed a heavy sack from her back. I thought of Jesus' parable of the prodigal son found in the fifteenth chapter of the gospel of Luke. When a weary son came back home after squandering his inheritance, his father did not punish the young man for his wrongdoing, but rather celebrated his return. As I gazed upon the young woman, tears welling up in my eyes, I realized that she was participating in a sort of homecoming, as well. I had no idea where she had been, but in light of God's grace, I knew that it didn't matter. God, and only God, had the power to transform the wreckage of the young woman's life into a masterpiece. A verse that feeds my soul when I feel caught in my own catastrophe came to mind: "And we know that in all things God works for the good of those who love him, who have been called according to his purpose" (Romans 8:28).

Homecoming—a process in which we may all take part if we are willing—willing to face the reality of our vulnerability and dependence. And the opportunity imposes no limits, but rather serves as a boundless source of grace for what has been, what is, and what will be. In receiving God's invitation to the path of peace, we find freedom in the fact that our very lives are not our own. Even though I didn't know the young woman's story, her mere being spoke this truth to me. Little did she know that in her weakness I saw God's strength, that in her fear I saw God's courage, that in her shame I saw God's acceptance, that in her desire I saw God's provision.

When the young woman returned to her seat, she sat crying with her face planted in her hands, occasionally looking up with a smile of bittersweet hope. I wondered if she was reflecting on the fact that she was much more than a pregnant unwed teenager; she was God's precious one. How comforting the truth is when we are willing to receive it.

As my husband and I got up to leave after the closing hymn, I longed to give my fellow sojourner a hug. I not only wanted to comfort her, but also myself, as I, too, yearn for my own homecoming. I sensed that God was using another one of His broken children to speak hope to me, to invite me into His arms. Following the Spirit's leading, I approached the young woman and gently touched her on the shoulder. She looked up at me and smiled. "You have blessed me more than you know, Dear One," I said, my words seeming to flow right out of me without a thought.

"Thank you," she graciously replied, as her tender smile exploded into a firecracker of sorts. Another outpouring of tears followed, accentuating her sparkling display as opposed to extinguishing it. As we embraced each other, I found myself somehow surprised by her response. "Shouldn't she be saying 'Really?' in disbelief, or 'Oh, you're too kind!'? " I thought to myself. But then I realized that the young woman's humility enabled her to see beyond her own pity. She appeared to see herself as she was—God's own—and invited me to do the same.

7

Letting Go
to Keep from Falling Apart

"Martha Claxton, Baptist, Oncology, Pastoral Support Requested," the referral card stated. As usual, I had little idea what kind of situation I was walking into. Was she gasping for her last breaths of air, did she simply long for a good listener, was she seeking a miraculous cure, or did she just want a Bible . . . ? The possible scenarios were endless, but the familiar feeling of vulnerability tempered by the knowledge of God's guiding presence accompanied them all. My own vulnerability and God's presence— what I used to see as mutually exclusive, I now experience as inseparable.

Not ready, but willing, I made my way to the Oncology Center. Mrs. Claxton's door loudly greeted me with a neon orange "ALL VISITORS MUST WEAR GOWN AND GLOVES BEFORE ENTERING" sign. I hate wearing protective garb, as it serves as another facilitator of the isolation I assume many patients already feel. The Martian uniform would have to do, however, for apparently the umpteenth round of chemo was taking its toll on Mrs. Claxton's immune system.

Mrs. Claxton welcomed me with a warm smile and an enthusiastic hello. Her kindness put me at ease. "I'm so glad you came, Chaplain. You know, my faith is all I got right now," she said, seemingly anxious to get right down to business. "Pull up a seat." I dragged the heavy metal black chair over from the corner and sat down next to her bedside. "That one's more comfortable," she offered, pointing to the large green recliner in the opposite corner. "That's okay," I assured her. "I'm already quite comfortable here with you." I smiled in return, wanting her to know that her hospitable spirit had done far more than any chair could do.

I couldn't help but immediately notice that the smooth black skin that graced the fifty-eight-year-old woman's face was a sharp contrast to the callous crust that enveloped the rest of her body. She sat perched on the bedside, repeatedly scratching patches of hardened and cracked skin. "My nerves have been so bad," she quickly related. "This skin is just too much. It's driving me crazy."

"It sounds like you're really uncomfortable," I reflected, not knowing what was worse, her physical or mental pain. Perhaps they were indistinguishable.

"Yes, I am miserable," she continued. "Last night, my skin was so bad that I had to bring a garbage can over to throw away all of the peel on my sheets." She shook her head shamefully, as if the condition was somehow her own fault. Just like her cancer-infested blood, her skin was now attacking and destroying her instead of protecting and nurturing her.

"What does all that skin peeling off mean to you?" I queried, seeking to dig deeper than her surface scratching. I sensed that Mrs. Claxton's skin condition suggested a lot more to her than a need for additional steroid cream.

"It means I'm falling apart," she stated bluntly, seemingly surprised by her own frankness. She looked up at me briefly, then returned her attention to the ceaseless scratching.

"*Falling apart . . .*" I repeated, uncertain of what to do with these heavy words. They collapsed into the air around us like bricks from an imploded building.

"But my faith, it really helps me," she said, returning to the safety of optimism. The truth was too scary to face head-on. Each itch that needed to be scratched, each glance in the full-length bathroom mirror already served as a constant reminder of her horrifying reality. Yes, faith was easier to talk about. Like a lighthouse glowing across stormy seas, it gave Mrs. Claxton the hope that her doctors could not.

"What is your experience of God through all this?" I asked, wondering how she felt amid the leukemia that seemed to be progressing as fiercely as a summer forest fire.

"He's testing me," she replied.

The response to my question was a familiar one, as many patients have said the same thing to me. "Oh, God's just testing me, seeing how much I can handle," they say in various ways, as if God isn't aware of our limits already, as if God's faithfulness depends on our own striving might.

"I just gotta be *stronger,* gotta hold on *tighter,*" Mrs. Claxton continued. She clenched her fists with the same vigor that her words suggested.

"What would happen if you let go?" I proposed. Mrs. Claxton looked at me as if I'd come from the psychiatric ward. "Huh?" I could hear her proclaiming inside her head. "What kind of crazy idea is that?" I sensed that my question needed clarification.

"I don't mean letting go of your *faith.* I mean letting go of your *might,*" I explained.

"Hmm . . ." she responded in deep thought. As we sat in silent contemplation, it occurred to me that I was proposing a way of life that eludes me on a daily basis. Constantly I give over to God what I know that only He can handle, yet immediately take it back again, as if my own fleeting efforts will bring to me the peace for which my heart thirsts. I wasn't just talking to Mrs. Claxton; I was also talking to myself.

"Oh, this skin is just too much!" Mrs. Claxton broke the silence, grumbling at her body's lifelong coat as if it were no longer a part of her. "I'm going to call the nurse." She hastily searched the rumpled sheets for the call button. It was clear to me that my proposal of letting go had hit too close to home for further consideration. She had already been stripped of nearly everything she had control over; why would she want to relinquish it all?

Aware that the nurse would enter momentarily, I asked Mrs. Claxton if she would like to have a prayer. "Oh, yes. I can never get enough prayer," she accepted. Bowing our heads, I offered my hand and invited the Holy Spirit to do the rest. Even though I didn't have a life-threatening illness, I was reminded that I, too, needed to depend on God in all things. I, too, needed to let go. With such divine guidance, words of my prayer flowed like warm honey, sweet and nourishing to our hungry hearts.

Not to my surprise, God brought forth through prayer what my own words alone could not: a heart whose brokenness now gave way for the Light to shine inside of it. Mrs. Claxton's eyes erupted with tears, and we embraced in an intimate hug, her body hanging on to mine like fruit on a vine. God has a way of doing that—of bringing us to a place of dependence and vulnerability so that He can indwell in us completely with His loving presence. Yes, vulnerability and God's presence: opposites on the surface that I find are really one in the heart.

8

Fertile Ground

Mr. Stark wanted to die. His doctors were willing to accommodate his wish, for after three years of endless suffering, his prognosis was dismal. The fifty-five-year-old man had received a lung transplant that didn't take, leaving him victim to countless infections. In and out of the hospital he would come and go, each time appearing a little more emaciated, a little paler, and a little more depressed. Finally, he had decided that the battle for a life of suffering was no longer worth the fight.

Maureen, the nurse who had cared for him throughout the course of his multiple admissions, called with the referral. "I don't want him to die alone," she said, knowing that the successful artist had virtually no family and only a couple of faithful friends who had not yet arrived. I headed up to the ward, sensing that Maureen was just as in need of pastoral care as was the patient for whom she cared so deeply.

I found Mr. Stark lying in bed, rapidly gasping for the air that seemed to elude his every inhalation. Each breath sounded like the squeal of a clogged vacuum cleaner. The doctors had removed the ventilator earlier that day upon his request, and then they had pumped him with megadoses of morphine for the dark night ahead. It was hard to imagine that the morphine was easing Mr. Stark's pain, as giant dollops of sweat dripped from his forehead with each labored gasp. In another sense, however, it was apparent that the suffering man had let go, moving from a place of battle and pain to a place of surrender and rest. As I reflected on his willingness to enter such a state of vulnerability, I realized that Mr. Stark was stronger than he appeared, full of a courageous trust that even a world-class triathlete is not guaranteed.

As we sat together, waiting in the uncertainty of whatever was to
come, I held Mr. Stark's clammy hand and stroked his wet brow with
a tissue. Before I knew it I was humming "Amazing Grace." The
gentle hymn coming from inside my mouth took me by surprise, and
I briefly hesitated, asking myself, "Where did that come from?" But
then my question quickly dissolved, needing no answer, only the
Spirit's tender confirmation inside for me to continue.

Mesmerized by the melody that had settled on my lips, I failed to
notice that Maureen had entered the room and was standing quietly
behind me. "I think it's nice that you sing to him," she murmured,
tenderly acquiring my attention. The nurse then took a seat at the
opposite side of the bed, and gazed solemnly at Mr. Stark with a
nostalgic grin on her face. I had no idea what she was thinking, only
that her thoughts were coming straight from her heart.

"He was such a special man," she began, speaking slowly with a
bittersweet sense of resolution. Mr. Stark was still alive, but Maureen was grieving the loss of the man as she knew him. "I have
cared for him for three years, you know. We became good friends
during all those admissions. I hate to see him go, but I know it's
what he wanted." I just listened, trying my best to provide a place
for her thoughts to be received.

"He was lonely all his life," she continued. "He struggled with
severe depression. It's so sad. He said he never allowed himself an
intimate relationship because he was so afraid of what people would
think."

At first Maureen's words confused me. "What do you mean he
was afraid what people would think?" I thought to myself. Then it
became clear to me that the single man was probably gay, and that
he had lived a life of fear and confusion about his sexuality. As I sat
there holding Mr. Stark's hand, my heart swelled with compassion,
for I often feel lonely, too. The feeling manifests itself in an incredi-
ble longing that can never be completely satisfied, as if I am float-.
ing in space millions of miles away from home. Unlike Mr. Stark,
however, I have my husband, my lover and soul mate, with whom I
can share my pain. While my dear one here on earth can never
completely fulfill my deepest desires, he encourages me with
blessed glimpses of the communion that is to come. I could only

hope that Mr. Stark had enjoyed such togetherness in some way here on earth.

I do not know what to think about homosexuality. There are some who say that the behavior is condemned by God, quoting the numerous scriptures that speak against it. Others contend that, just like committed heterosexual relationships, committed homosexual relationships can be another avenue for expressing divine love to each other. I avoid taking any stance, perhaps in an attempt to run away from what God himself may speak to me about it in my heart. Or maybe I sit on the fence as a result of my own insecurity, fearing the disapproval of those with whom I discuss the topic. In any case, however, my uncertainty is undergirded by God's call to love, the only lasting hope in which we can all find refuge with one another.

In the midst of my thoughts, Maureen glanced at her watch and stood up. "I have to go," she said with a sigh that suggested both disappointment and relief. "My daughter has a soccer game." She then leaned over Mr. Stark, kissed him on the forehead, and whispered, "Good-bye, Tim. I love you." Her few words couldn't have been more sufficient.

"Thanks for being here," she said, looking over at me. "I just didn't want him to be alone, especially since that's how he's lived his whole life."

"I can see you really care about him," I replied. Deep down, I wondered if Maureen had found a sense of pleasure and purpose in offering to Mr. Stark what she herself also longed for—a true friend. This is a familiar scenario for those who work in helping professions, including myself: we seek to give what we long to receive.

As we both gazed at Mr. Stark, it occurred to me that the wheezing man was far from being alone. Even if we were not there, he would always be in the hearts of Maureen, myself, and all those whose lives he had unknowingly touched. Furthermore, having surrendered his life, he would soon be in the company of the One who so freely gives new life to all those who are willing to receive it.

"It's wonderful to know that he soon won't feel alone anymore," I reflected aloud with a smile on my face.

"Well, I don't know about that," Maureen responded. "I don't know about what happens after death." Her statement surprised me,

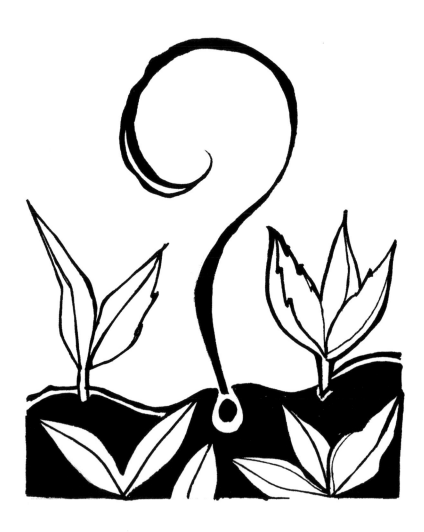

as I had not thought of my words as being objectionable, especially since Maureen herself had called for a chaplain. I immediately learned yet again, however, that my experience of God cannot be assumed onto others', only offered in its proper timing.

At first, I didn't know quite what to say in response to Maureen, for her words of uncertainty left me speechless. Part of me wanted to retort with a thorough explanation of the gospel of Jesus Christ, the message of love and grace that has forever changed my life. But then I realized that Maureen did not need my answers, but rather a place to bring her questions. In fact, in her willingness to expose her incertitude, she encouraged me to be open to listening for God's voice in my life all the more instead of clinging desperately to what has been revealed to me thus far.

"Your uncertainty is very becoming," I finally replied, realizing that it was only in such a state of emptiness and openness that God could fill her.

"What do you mean?" she asked, seemingly surprised by my observation. I wondered if anyone had ever affirmed her searching instead of trying to stuff destinations down her throat.

"I mean that your uncertainty makes way for fertile ground," I responded. Maureen continued to stand at the foot of Mr. Stark's bed, seeming to digest what she had just heard.

"In fact, maybe that's what Mr. Stark needed in you," I continued, looking up at Maureen with a smile.

"Yeah," she laughed. "And I think that's what I needed in him, too."

9

Blessed Are the Poor in Spirit

"I happy!" Ms. May announced with a friendly giggle. The thirty-eight-year-old woman with Down's syndrome was undoubtedly one of the most content patients I have ever met in the hospital, perhaps even one of the most agreeable persons I have ever met anywhere. She sat hoisted up in bed on top of a pile of pillows, looking as though her beaming smile actually had the power to spring her right through the ceiling. With her eyes fixed to the Smurfs on the television, she appeared oblivious to the wire leads pulling at her chest and the beeps emanating from the heart monitor. Even though she was sick, she was a stark contrast to the other faces of misery that I had visited earlier that morning.

Ms. May is not the first person I have ever met with Down's syndrome, and I doubt she will be the last. For this I am thankful, as I find that many who share her so-called handicap are actually blessed with a boundless ability to live the present moment to the fullest. Unlike those of us who can hide within the confines of our minds, Ms. May and others with mental handicaps seem to be able to trust that what is happening now is worth their undivided attention, not clinging to the past for a sense of security, nor racing ahead into the future for an escape from present anxiety. Yes, Ms. May could worry about impending heart failure, or she could regret the fact that her life was void of any children or professional degrees. But, instead, she focused on what was at hand—watching the Smurfs with a hospital chaplain—seeming to leave every other concern in the hands of the God who had led her thus far. Little did Ms. May know that the carefree attitude she so naturally possessed was the very one that eludes me on a daily basis.

Had I known that Ms. May was retarded, I confess that I may have not chosen to knock on her door. Frozen in the deception of my own capacities, I may have reasoned that such a person wasn't worth my time. "Well, we wouldn't be able to have a meaningful conversation," I can hear myself reasoning, as if our minds were the only things we had to offer each other. Stripped of any sophisticated thoughts and complex emotions, Ms. May had something different to give: herself, her heart, her very being.

Fortunately, for my sake and hers, Ms. May's joyful response to my knock gave me no choice but to enter. "Hi!" she burst out, with a gigantic smile that exposed all of her teeth. I tried my best to return the enthusiastic greeting, one that I am not accustomed to seeing in the presence of hospital patients. However, Ms. May seemed to know that despite her sickness, her life still had something to celebrate. She waved her hands in excitement, then placed them on the sides of her face, providing a perfect frame for her plump cheeks and jubilant grin.

As I introduced myself, Ms. May just looked up at me, seeming to see right through my words. The message I wanted to communicate already seemed apparent to her: "I'm here for you." She immediately pointed up to the television, as if to invite me on a picnic to taste her favorite goodies. I accepted her offer, taking a seat at her bedside and turning my eyes to the screen. Frantically running through the woods, Papa Smurf bumped into a tree and flew through the air. Ms. May giggled with delight and looked over at me, shrugging her shoulders and shaking her head as if she needed yet another way to express her joy. I joined in the laughter, not in response to Papa Smurf's clumsy bouncing body, but because of the simple bliss that Ms. May seemed to have released in me.

As we sat watching cartoons together, it occurred to me that in Ms. May's presence, I felt a peace that was not of the world, around which my life so regularly rotates. All of my abilities and possessions that I so frequently pursue for a sense of security suddenly dimmed in comparison to the contentment in which Ms. May appeared so firmly grounded. A familiar passage of scripture came to life in my mind: ". . . God chose the weak things of the world to shame the strong, . . . so that no man may boast before him" (1Corinthians 1:27, 29). Yes, Ms. May exuded a peace not dictated by the circumstance of the moment, but by the very existence of the moment itself; not dominated by what she had, but by the fact that she had anything at all. A peace grounded in trust—simple and pure, like an infant's at a mother's breast. No, Ms. May could not *do* much, but she could *be* much—for me and for many. In her very weakness, she invited those around her back to their hearts, back to their homes, back to the present, back to the place where God speaks. She reminded me of who I was, who she was, who we all are: children in the palms of God's hands.

My reveries were temporarily interrupted when the nurse suddenly entered. "The doctor wants me to put some 'dig'* in your IV; okay, dear?" Ms. May's face lit up yet again at the sight of Beth, one of the many nurses who frequently looked as overworked as she really was. She quickly flicked the bubbles out of the syringe, repeatedly wiping from her line of vision the strands of hair that had escaped her ponytail. I wondered if any of her other patients were as glad to see her in her frazzled state, syringe in hand. I didn't think so. In fact, Ms. May's tender spirit was probably just as therapeutic to Beth as Beth's vigilant nursing care was to her.

As Beth slowly injected the heart medication, Ms. May tensed with pain, sensing its characteristic sting. She tightly gripped my offered hand, seeming to know that pain, as well as joy, was something to be shared. Tears rolled down her cheeks, serving their analgesic purpose with each released drop. It was hard to believe that just a moment prior, Ms. May had been engulfed in a wave of smiles and laughter. Happy or sad, her emotions shone freely from the window of her soul, pure and genuine, not distorted by pride.

Ms. May calmed down within a few minutes, her tears drying as quickly as they had first poured out. "I'm sorry, Ms. May," Beth apologized, gently stroking her back. "I wish it didn't sting so bad like that." Ms. May just looked up at her, appearing to see the nurse's show of compassion rather than the painful shot she represented. She donned her familiar smile that seemed to put anyone at ease who laid eyes on her. "I okay," Ms. May said, opening her arms to welcome Beth. The two embraced in a joyful hug, inviting me to join in.

Ms. May bid me farewell in the same cheerful manner as she had greeted me. As I waved good-bye, my entire being radiated with

---

*"Dig" is medical slang for digoxin, a heart medication. It is pronounced "dĭj."

genuine warmth. It was a warmth only possible in the presence of Divine Acceptance, a presence that makes its most secure home in the hearts of those who are rejected. Certainly, Ms. May had been rejected, cast aside by a society that values what we do and not who we are. But in her very debility, she was eternally accepted. And as a result, through the cracks of her broken heart, God's love shone forth like a heavenly searchlight, piercing the darkness of all courageous enough to welcome its healing light.

10

Not Religious, but Real

"If God is so all powerful," Mr. Davis grumbled, "then why doesn't he just come down right this minute and introduce himself to me?" At first, the thirty-six-year-old man's question struck me as irreverent. "How dare he challenge God," I thought to myself. But then I realized that Mr. Davis's question was not unique to his thoughts; in fact, it had crossed my mind more than once in the past. I, too, have wondered why God doesn't do what makes perfect sense to me, especially during difficult times. "You know, God," I remember thinking as I lay curled up in a fetal position in my college dorm room, suffering my third year of bowel disease, "why don't you just cure me? It would be so glorifying to you, and I would have so much more energy to serve you!" Looking back now, I see that if I had understood God's reasoning at that point, my faith would have been deprived of fertile soil in which to grow.

Unlike Mr. Davis, however, I often felt compelled to hide my feelings and doubts from God and others, as if they couldn't see the real me lurking behind the camouflage of a carefully constructed mask. "God, I thank you that you are going to use this illness in my life in some way," I remember bitterly trying to convince myself. It occurred to me that perhaps Mr. Davis was more willing to be honest with himself than I was. Yes, this straight-talking man who claimed no creed indeed had his own brand of humility to offer.

Mr. Davis had been through a lot over the past year, and his future was anything but certain. He had just been diagnosed with a terminal heart condition that would require a transplant for long-term survival. To top things off, his wife had recently left him for another man. Mr. Davis's world was falling apart. The heart that pumped his blood, the wife who had been his intimate companion, the hunting and fishing that had turned his weekends into retreats, the spicy meals that he had enjoyed preparing: all these things were no longer realities, but only events that he had never before recognized as true gifts.

Mr. Davis's story spewed from his lips like water from a fire hydrant. He spoke quickly, in a bazaar matter-of-fact sort of way. It didn't seem to matter that *I* was listening, only that *someone* was. His unshaven chin was littered with specks of dried blood from the central line that had been inserted into the jugular vein in his neck; his greasy hair was projecting in every direction; and his body was held taut by multiple intravenous lines protruding from his bruised skin. Mr. Davis looked like a modern-day Job. Perplexed and ragged, he sat cross-legged in the middle of his elevated bed, clinging to the pile of flimsy sheets that covered his lap. He looked as though he wanted to leap off the bed and run out of the hospital, but was restrained by the realization that his real-life nightmare would follow him wherever he went.

"You know, my mother sure would enjoy talking to you," Mr. Davis suddenly blurted, bypassing the serious course of his words. I just nodded in response, wondering where this detour would take us. "She's very religious," he continued, anxious to turn the subject away from himself. "She made me go to church when I was a kid, and I think that's why I still don't like it." As this third person mysteriously entered the picture, I imagined a bony, iron-handed woman with a stern voice saying, "Get ready for church, young man!" I wondered if this is how Mr. Davis saw me. Indeed, such an association would place me in a less than desirable position. I wanted to attract him to God, not repel him.

"I can see why you wouldn't like church if you were forced to go as a child," I replied, attempting to realign myself with Mr. Davis. His candid approach to his feelings about religion caught me off guard, yet at the same time, they aroused in me a newfound regard for his rare breed of sincerity. I thought of the numerous patients I see who enthusiastically proclaim God's goodness in the midst of dire circumstances, denying the pain that humanity invokes. "Oh, I'm just praising the Lord for all these wonderful doctors and nurses," I recall a bubbly woman exclaiming between cries of pain from a recently amputated foot. No, Mr. Davis didn't have much to say to God. But at least if he ever did, his words would likely be genuine. At least if he ever sought God, his search would be sincere. Mr. Davis wasn't religious, but he was real.

Our conversation continued, waxing and waning from the superficial to the serious. Mr. Davis seemed to boldly confront the gravity of his situation, yet only for a moment at a time, as if dipping his toes into a hot bath. The water of life would scald him if he jumped in. He seemed to know on a level that he was not yet willing to acknowledge, however, that he would have to take a swim eventually.

"Well, if you ever see a healthy two-hundred-pound man on the side of the street, tell him to step in front of a car so I can have his heart," Mr. Davis joked. "You'll have to excuse me. I have a morbid sense of humor," he continued, shaking his head with a snicker. We both smiled and chuckled at his joke that had somehow served as a sort of refuge from reality, not just for him, but also for me. At times I wondered who was more overwhelmed by the situation—him or me?

As our laughter subsided, Mr. Davis looked up at me, raising his open hands with a sense of resignation. "Well, Chaplain," he said. "I figure that if there's a God, He can relate to my situation and He knows what I need."

I responded with a humbled grin, recognizing that Mr. Davis understood the nature of the Mercy he couldn't yet identify. But upon further evaluation, it became clear to me that he lacked the sense of responsibility necessary to respond to God's call for relationship. He seemed to want to be raised up without lifting his hand. Now that his life was falling apart, I wondered if Mr. Davis would have the courage to reach out to the One who called his name, to the One who would be strength in his weakness, light in his darkness, peace in his terror. Or would his feelings about the rotten hand life had dealt him only serve to devour his heart like a creeping mildew?

The next time I saw Mr. Davis was several weeks after a successful heart transplant. He was just getting into the shower. "Oh, hi, Gretchen," he said. "It's nice of you to come by. Can you come back after I've had a chance to clean up?" I told him how wonderful it was to see him doing well, agreed to return later, and then headed back to the nurses' station. Little did I know then that that was the last time I would ever see Mr. Davis.

"Yes, he died the next day," the nurse had said. "He got into some really bad rhythms." I felt like the wind had been knocked out of me, as the news left me speechless. I stood paralyzed for a few seconds, and then began to cry. I wept not tears of anger or tears of regret, but, rather, tears of deep sadness. I grieved the loss of a man who possessed an honesty that would have made faith real, a man who caused me to examine the sincerity of my own thoughts and feelings. He appealed to the hidden rebel in me, the person who longs to question all the "shoulds" and listen more intently to all the "coulds." Did I encourage Mr. Davis to reach out to the Loving One he already sensed was there, to seek the God who wasn't confined to his childhood memories? I cannot say; actually, I fear not. But I take great comfort in the fact that the One who gave him life and took it away knows his heart, and that's all that really matters.

11

The Man Without a Nose

Mr. Catalino didn't have a nose. Or at least the bump on the center of his face didn't look like a nose. "They took it off to get the cancer," his wife said. "And then they put skin from his forehead on it to cover it up." I listened intently, commanding myself not to gag. Mr. Catalino looked as if someone had torn off his nose, then put a malformed hunk of bloody clay in its place. Pieces of gauze protruded from both sides, attempting to arrest the bleeding that had worsened overnight.

The couple from North Carolina had requested earlier that day that a chaplain stop by. I accepted the referral immediately, preferring such visits to random ones because in them I know that I am at least wanted. In any case, I don't think Mr. and Mrs. Catalino got what they expected. "You're an awfully young chaplain," the sixty-two-year-old man remarked, both adults scanning me up and down several times. Their response to my initial presence was nothing new, for it wasn't the first time I have experienced it. As hard as I try with lipstick and "grown-up clothes," my petite frame frequently evokes an image more like a candy striper's than that of a hospital chaplain. However, I am learning that when I let God's spirit of love and humility dwell freely within me, my outward appearance flows naturally along with it, leaving behind any of the unnecessary assumptions or stereotypes. No, I cannot try to be someone I am not; I can only be continually transformed and made into the person God designed for His purposes.

"Yes, I do look young for my age," I acknowledged. The three of us just smiled and laughed, perpetuating the awkwardness that accompanies many of my initial visits. Sometimes I wonder if I will ever be as relaxed and discerning as many of my mentors appear to be in similar situations, or if my discomfort and uncertainty are an inevitable part of being a chaplain. Probably both. In fact, I am coming to realize that it is only in my discomfort that God provides me with His ease, that it is only in my uncertainty that God gives me His discernment.

"Well, it looks like you've been through a lot," I began, anxious to change the subject from my youthfulness to something more relevant.

"Yes, I have," Mr. Catalino agreed, pointing to an empty chair at the bedside. As I sat down, he shared a lengthy lament of his cancer and recent surgery. After months of headaches, blurry vision, and bloody noses, a tumor the size of a golf ball behind his sinuses had showed up on the MRI scan. The doctors were worried about the pressure it was exerting on his brain, what function it would declare war on next, and where its poisonous protrusions would invade in the months to come. Surgery was the only treatment option. And with the cancer, his nose would have to go, too.

"I just hope they got all the cancer," he pleaded, rescuing a teardrop from falling into the bloody crater between his eyes. "Every time I look at my face in the mirror, I see it, I see *the cancer*." Even if the surgeons had eradicated the tumor, I realized that for Mr. Catalino, he would always have cancer. His nose, or lack thereof, marked his face like a scarlet letter: a constant reminder of his vulnerability, and a freakish defect for everyone to point at and criticize. "Oh, gross; look at that man's face," I recalled my own thoughts upon first meeting Mr. Catalino. "He looks like the Elephant Man." Sadly, I knew my thoughts would be others' thoughts, and even the cruel words of some.

Mr. Catalino pulled up the tray from his bedside table and peered into the little mirror tucked inside of it. As soon as he caught a glimpse of his horrifying reflection, he slammed the device back into the compartment as if it wasn't meant for his use. Bursting into a frenzy of half-restrained sobs, he carefully buried his face in a handful of crumpled sheets.

Mrs. Catalino draped her arm around her husband, she, too, shedding tears of sorrow. Mr. Catalino leaned slightly toward her, resting his shoulder on her chest, seeming to trust that she was a safe place for him to bring his aching heart. I noticed how through-

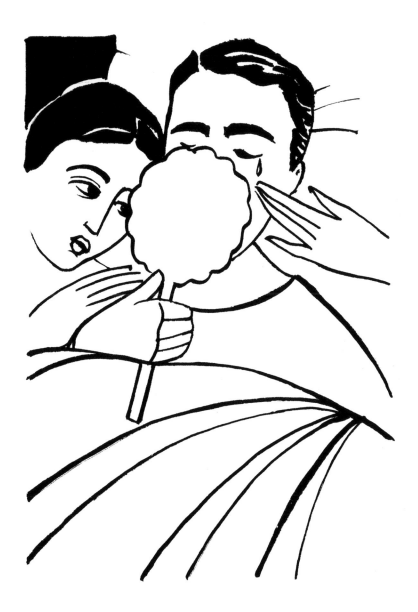

out the visit, the couple attended to each other with the ease of two soaring eagles. Their interactions reminded me of the oneness of two joined rings, always together to varying degrees, but never the same.

I sat speechless, sensing that the moment required my silence more than my words. Part of me wanted to rescue Mr. Catalino from what appeared to be a pit of grief, but deep down, I knew that the painful place in which he found himself was also a sort of refuge for him at that time. It was not a place that he wanted to go, but a place he needed to go, and it was my honor to be able to accompany him there.

After a few minutes had passed, I slowly reached out and lightly touched my fingers to one of the grieving man's exposed cheeks. By reaching out to the very source of his pain, as repulsive as it was, I wanted him to know that *he* was still lovable. Yes, his nose was unsightly, but it was *his* nose. And yes, it rudely declared "cancer!" every time he looked into the mirror, but this gentle man with genuine emotions could not be reduced to a disease.

The longer the three of us sat still and silent, the more pronounced Mr. Catalino's sorrow became, like a freight train picking up momentum with each chug. Finally, his tears ceased as if his well of grief had temporarily run dry.

After he calmed down, he slowly raised his head and gazed with bleary eyes into mine. A gentle grin settled upon his lips, transforming his deformed face into a message of peace rather than one of agony. I struggled to remain silent, sensing that the message of love and acceptance I longed to put into words had already been heard.

After several minutes of silence, Mr. Catalino closed his eyes and took a slow deep breath, as if the air itself had a healing quality. "I think I'm going to be okay," he declared. With his words came an exhalation of peaceful resignation. He seemed to know that even though his malformed nose and the cancer it represented would be with him wherever he went, so also would God. And God was bigger than these things that attempted to threaten his very being; in fact, God was the source of his being.

"I'd say that God thinks you're going to be okay, too," I replied, turning our attention to the Presence who had been there all along.

The three of us laughed, acknowledging the reality that had ironically become so apparent in the midst of tragedy.

Mr. Catalino was certain to face many difficult experiences of rejection and vulnerability in the days ahead, but I hoped that he would remember then that it was during such times that he also could discover and rediscover his own inherent preciousness to God. Yes, to God, the One who made his nose, the One who made *him*.

12

Called to Wait

On the surface, my visit with Mrs. Hendrix appeared routine and uneventful: a simple "Hello. How are you doing?" followed by a brief prayer. However, upon further reflection I have learned that our time together was truly momentous. It was pregnant with God's presence, a presence that made itself known in stillness instead of motion, in waiting versus activity.

Mrs. Hendrix was the first of three referrals I had received that morning. Anxious to "get them done," I headed up to the ward with my own unconscious agenda: to come, to save, and to leave as quickly as possible. My destructive mind-set left God out of the picture, making way for my will and not His to be done. But even in the midst of my pride, God seemed to cut through my defenses, gradually transforming my time with Mrs. Hendrix into a retreat instead of a project.

I knocked on the elderly woman's door, and was welcomed by a feeble voice. "Come in, dear," she whispered. The tender way in which she called me into her room made me feel as if we already knew each other, as if she so wisely saw me as a fellow child of God instead of just a chaplain. Her hospitable spirit seemed to disarm me in part, and my frantic plans suddenly took a backseat to the moment at hand.

According to the nurse, Mrs. Hendrix had been in and out of the hospital for over a year with multiple health problems: kidney disease, cellulitis, heart trouble, diabetes. The list seemed endless. It was no longer a matter of curing Mrs. Hendrix, but of finding ways to make her more comfortable. Even this was beginning to appear to be too much to ask.

After I introduced myself, Mrs. Hendrix shared how glad she was that I had come. "Oh, how wonderful. You're here," she whispered in as joyful a voice as her fragile state would allow. At first, her gratitude left me speechless, for I hadn't even done anything for her yet. But then I realized that by simply coming, I had given her a tangible form of the communion her heart longed for. She sat rigidly in bed like a stick doll, offering an ever-so-slight smile between grimaces of pain.

"So how are you doing?" I asked, eager to get on with the visit, as if it weren't already where it needed to be. Actually, the answer to my question had already been offered in her facial expressions of pain, and in her few words and the weak voice in which they were delivered. But I simply wasn't listening.

"I can't talk much," she replied, kindly pinpointing my impatient spirit that was blinding me from God's guidance. Looking back, I now see that through Mrs. Hendrix's inability to speak, God was calling me to give up my own speech and become like her: an open place for God to respond. Yes, God was calling me to do what He so willingly does for us: wait.

"I have . . . bad kidneys," she slowly muttered, probably more for my sake than hers. "And . . . they're putting in . . . a pacemaker. . . . The doctor will be coming by . . . with my husband." After the long string of words, she let out a gasp of relief.

"You don't need to talk," I offered, attempting to repair the damage of my unnecessary inquiry. I felt somewhat ashamed, recognizing that my desire to be in control of the visit had led her to a place of torture rather than comfort. Yes, in a dire attempt to conquer my primary fear of being out of control, I had hurt not only Mrs. Hendrix, but also myself. Deep down, I knew it was time for me to let go, to stay in the uncomfortable uncertainty, to let God take the next step, to wait.

Waiting. In her very inability to do anything for herself, Mrs. Hendrix seemed to have received the ability to wait for what God would do for her. She no longer could care for herself and others, so she had no other choice than to let others care for her. Mrs. Hendrix so courageously occupied the very place that I spend much of my energy running away from. She waited for the doctor, she waited for her husband, she waited for the pain medication to take effect, she waited for her wounds to heal, she waited for the lunch tray to come, she waited for the nurse to respond to the call button. She waited. And yes, it was a painful waiting, but in her absence of striving, I also sensed it was a hopeful waiting, a waiting that did not require words, only listening; a waiting that did not require movement, only a willingness to be at home.

As we sat in the fullness of the silence, I sensed God's active presence among us. How revealing it was to consider that God's purposes were being accomplished in both of us, not in what we were *doing*, but in what we were *allowing to be done* unto ourselves. To be truly present in such a place of openness was freeing, like standing on a mountaintop on a clear day, viewing the endless landscape. At the same time, it was frightening, for to be a true recipient of whatever God would have for me is difficult. It requires a willingness to wait, to trust, to surrender, to be open and empty, to be in preparation rather than destination, to become dependent. In short, it requires a willingness to become that which we already are: God's very own.

In the midst of my thoughts, I suddenly was reminded of the fact that it was Holy Week, a time in the church calendar that couldn't be more appropriate for the situation at hand. Gazing at Mrs. Hendrix, I thought of Jesus in Gethsemane before the crucifixion. In his agony, he prayed and opened himself completely to his Father's will; he waited for God and at the same time waited for us: his betrayers. He didn't run away from the pain of the moment, as I so often do, but he remained faithful to it. And he didn't ask his disciples to do anything for him, only to be present with him. Would I, just as the disciples, choose to enter a slumber of sorts to gain some sort of control over the situation? Or, would I choose to be present with Mrs. Hendrix and find hope in the vulnerable place of waiting? A telling piece of scripture then came to mind, revealing to me the true desire of my heart. "I want to know Christ and the power of his resurrection and the fellowship of sharing in his sufferings, becoming like him in his death, and so, somehow, to attain to the resurrection from the dead" (Philippians 3:10). Yes, Easter was just around the corner, but not without Good Friday to prepare for its arrival.

After several moments of silence, Mrs. Hendrix proposed that we have a prayer together. I agreed, trying not to jump too quickly at the opportunity to act. "I just want to pray for the pain of the whole world," she offered, settling her head back into the pillow. Her request took me by surprise, as I was expecting her to include herself in prayer.

"What do you mean by everyone?" I inquired, wondering who exactly was behind her request. Again, I simply wasn't listening, for I would soon realize that Mrs. Hendrix *had* included herself in prayer, simply in another way: in the pain of all those around her. She seemed to know that she was not alone, that her experience was alive in all of humanity. In that way, I suspect that she felt my pain, too.

"I don't want to talk anymore," she finally said in response to my question, looking at me with the spirit of patience that seemed to have found its home in her. She seemed to trust that, at that moment, to try to explain to me what God already knew would be a futile endeavor.

I laughed quietly to myself, thanking God for the additional reminder through His faithful eighty-two-year-old servant. "When will I learn to just receive you, Lord? When will I learn to wait in the place of uncertainty?" I thought to myself. Before I could come up with my own answers, God saved me with His own. "You are learning," I heard the Voice inside of me say. Again, I learned that God was right there with me in my questions, and not in the place of answers that I so desperately seek.

—13—

Recollection

Mr. Jones had caught my eye as I was making rounds on the Cardiac Care Unit earlier that day. The elderly black man had been sitting up straight as a cornstalk in bed, his head protruding slightly forward so as to peer through the open doorway into the hall. Alert and watchful, he appeared as if he had been expecting my visit all day long.

I awkwardly knocked on his door, knowing full well that I already had his complete attention. He nodded abruptly, and I entered the room, feeling drawn by both my curiosity and a sense of obligation.

"Hello, Mr. Jones. My name is Gretchen TenBrook and I'm a chaplain here at the hospital," I began. My usual introduction seemed to augment his vigilant state, as he suddenly began jerking his legs anxiously under the covers. Now that I was in his room, he seemed to look at everything around him except me. I couldn't decide whether he was nervous or excited, perhaps both. Part of me wanted to ask him about his peculiar demeanor, but then I realized that bringing attention to it would only serve to suppress the thoughts and feelings behind it—thoughts and feelings that were yearning for a place to be expressed.

Despite Mr. Jones' somewhat erratic behavior, I sensed that he wanted me present. He seemed to want me just to be with him, just to listen to him. This didn't take me long to recognize; before I could even take a seat at his bedside, he started sharing with me a wealth of what seemed to be unrelated memories—about the artichokes on the farm and how they didn't taste like those "hot house" ones; about the poor boy with manure on his shoe and the rich boy wearing cologne who both thought each other stunk; about how he didn't want to kill the German who didn't want to kill him; about the dope on the streets and the grandchildren he had lost to it; about his lovely wife who had died in the same hospital in which he now lay; about how he got accused of something he didn't do. . . . Sometimes his recollections didn't make much sense. "How did he go from artichokes to World War II?" I thought to myself. But deep down, I knew it didn't matter. What mattered was that his stories were heard, and that I was there to receive them.

The stories flowed, and with them, I noticed that his anxious behaviors subsided. His legs ceased their restless twitching and his eyes quit their sporadic perusing. All of his senses now appeared to be calmly focused on the memories at hand, places and times that I suspected he had been longing to revisit in the genuine company of another for quite some time.

Although all of Mr. Jones' recollections were clothed in an alluring nostalgia, I sensed a sadness that seemed to emanate from them. "Things aren't the way they used to be," he had said several times. Like so many other elderly men and women I have met in my hospital ministry, Mr. Jones was mourning the multiple losses of his life: his wife, the food he used to enjoy on the farm, the innocence of his youth, the relationships he wished he had been able to nurture better, and now—his health. Mr. Jones was slowly losing control. "I just don't want to be a bother to anyone," he said, resisting the gradual departure of the independence that he most certainly had taken for granted in his younger years.

Nearly an hour had passed before I realized that I needed to close the visit. My attention had been fully extended and my ears were full of blessings. His mind had been fully emptied and his heart was full of peace. The gifts had been given and received, and now it was time to go.

I have always been taught not to stretch a visit out too long, for the patient's sake and for mine. For the patient—whose body is tired from trauma and tests, whose mind is weary from diagnoses and decisions, whose spirit is consumed with mixed feelings of hope and fear. For me—to preserve my own limited ability to concentrate and truly hear what patients are saying, with or without words. Yes, this work is exhausting at times. "You look tired today," I remember a patient telling me one afternoon. "Hmm . . . is this

God's way of showing me I need to get some rest?" I remember thinking to myself. I learn over and over again that the patients seem to minister to me just as much as I minister to them.

"Would you like to have a prayer before I leave, Mr. Jones?" I asked. The Baptist with the warm heart nodded in affirmation. "Do you mind if I hold your hand?" I queried. A smile settled on his face, as if he needed to be touched just as much as he needed to be listened to.

Mr. Jones and I bowed our heads, and I thanked God for this man and his life. My words seemed to flow out naturally, lacking the clumsiness that I feel all too often characterizes my prayers. The Spirit was at work; somehow God was feeding me with the words to say. Yet I have learned over time that even when the words don't come, I can still trust that all is well, for God still knows what the patients need and He still knows what I need. Whatever I pray or don't pray, God still *is*.

"All this we pray in Jesus' name," I closed. Mr. Jones squeezed my hand, sandwiching it between his two hands, which looked as tough as bear claws but felt as soft as worn leather. Suddenly, he rested his chin on his chest, and tears began to flow. His body shook silently with each sob. His weeping felt clean and healthy to me, as if it was making fertile ground for whatever was to come. It was relief for him. I could see it in his shoulders which no longer stood high and tense, but rested limp; I could see it in his legs which no longer jerked, but lay motionless; I could see it in his eyes which no longer wandered, but looked gently up at me.

"Thank you. God bless you, my child," he said quietly.

"It was my honor," I replied, feeling my smile extend from my lips to my toes. I was temporarily awed by how this man with a million stories had so richly blessed me. Yes, the gifts had been given and received.

"May I give you a hug?" I offered. Somehow this display of affection came naturally. I leaned over his elevated bed and we gently embraced. We were strangers, yet as close as two siblings in the family of God. My long thin hair got stuck on his scratchy, unshaven chin. We both laughed. And then he cried a little more. And God was there, in the fullness of all the emotions.

—14—

Faces of Grief

The referral from the Surgical ICU was urgent. Urgent—a word that made my heart skip a beat, for it implied that there was no time to prepare. But then again, I guess I can never be completely prepared for anything, a realization that I often revisit, inviting me to lean on God's guidance all the more.

Mr. Dixon, a fifty-something Muslim, was dying of end-stage AIDS, and according to the doctors, it didn't look as if his tired heart would beat much longer. As I read the information from the referral card, my mind was overtaken by a swarm of insecurity. "Oh, Lord, can't someone else take this one?" I pleaded inside my head. "I don't want to mess up this one. You don't want me, of all people! You want someone with experience . . ." Just like Moses, who out of his own insecurity presented God with multiple reasons why he thought he couldn't lead the Israelites out of bondage, I also searched for any excuse and came up empty. My plea for deliverance appeared unanswered, but in actuality God's silence spoke loudly. "Hush, my child. Go, for I am with you," I felt Him saying to me in my heart of hearts.

"Mr. Dixon is in room eleven," the nurse informed me as I arrived on the unit. "The wife, Mrs. Dixon, and the patient's sister, Gina, are down there," she said, pointing toward the conference room at the end of the hallway. I made my way down the corridor, passing rooms occupied by ailing patients and the big beeping and gasping machines that were keeping them alive. The intensive care units always present a certain paradox to me: the wonder of modern medicine alongside the tragedy of acute suffering. I often ponder who is being treated: the disease or the patient? Certainly the two share no common boundary.

As I entered the conference room I found the two African-American women sitting in the far corner in tears. They sat hunched over in their chairs like two floppy pillows. No sooner had I introduced myself to them, when Dr. Ulion walked into the room to explain the dire situation. With a stoic look on his face, he pulled up a chair.

"Mrs. Dixon, I'm afraid that I don't have any good news to tell you. Your husband is very sick, and there's not much more we can do." Dr. Ulion proceeded to explain the details of the predicament: Mr. Dixon's fluid-filled heart was no longer able to pump blood to his extremities, causing his kidneys and liver to fail; the blood supply to his brain was also minimal, suggesting that permanent damage would be imminent; his already compromised immune system couldn't fight the fungal infection in his blood; the ventilator was doing all his breathing for him; he wasn't responding to the megadoses of antibiotics and pressors;* his blood pressure was dropping and his heart rate rising, implying that his heart was rapidly failing. "There's about a two percent chance he will survive," Dr. Union stated bluntly after painting the complete grim scenario. He then confirmed the "Do Not Resuscitate" order written boldly on the front of Mr. Dixon's medical chart. The red DNR sticker reminded me of a "Dangerous Curve Ahead" road sign, suggesting imminent death was the most likely destination.

Mrs. Dixon and Gina exploded into yet deeper sobs, their cries not allowing them to come up with any verbal response to Dr. Ulion's report. The kind, yet straightforward physician seemed to understand that their grief would have to take precedence at least for a few minutes, and he left the room, agreeing to return with any additional updates. As I stroked the women's shoulders in an attempt to provide comfort, I sensed that for them Mr. Dixon had already died. Yes, he was still alive, but I suspected that the part of him they longed to save had just perished with the doctor's dreadful news. Even more, I wondered if the Keith they cherished in their hearts had begun disintegrating long ago, the AIDS virus eating away at his body like a multiplying parasite. My Spirit-led insight then mutated into mere curiosity: "How did Mr. Dixon get AIDS? Did Mrs. Dixon contract it from him? If so, how could she love

---

*Pressors are medications given intravenously to raise blood pressure.

him?" Such questions teased my desire to know, yet also served to remind me of my role: to comfort, not to inquire.

The two women's mourning was suddenly interrupted by the shriek of a small elderly black woman entering the room. "What's all this crying about?" she yelled. "It ain't gonna solve the problem! Man, I don't need this!" She then turned to me, boldly introducing herself. "Hi, I'm Mrs. Patricia Dixon, Keith's mother."

"Hi," I replied in half the volume. "My name is Gretchen Ten-Brook and I'm a chaplain."

"Well, praise the Lord Jesus you're here," she said, throwing her hands up into the air while pacing the room. Obviously she did not share her son's Islamic faith. Noting this fact, it occurred to me that ironically, this was the first time during the visit that I had thought about the specific faith traditions of the people to whom I was ministering. It became clear to me that in the midst of the tragedy, God's all-encompassing love was transcending any divisions we could make among ourselves.

"Maybe you can help *them!*" the old woman continued, pointing to her lamenting daughter and daughter-in-law. Part of me wanted to tell her that maybe she needed to cry, too, for in my experience tears are one of God's ways of getting our attention. They bring us closer to that very person, place, or thing we so deeply care about, as if each descending teardrop is proclaiming "Look, hear, for God speaks!" I am reminded of Jesus' reaction when Mary lamented to him that if he had been there earlier, her brother Lazarus would not have died. In response, "Jesus wept," the apostle John wrote in his gospel. "Then the Jews said, 'See how he loved him [Lazarus]!'" (John 11:35-36). Just like those of Jesus, Mrs. Dixon and Gina's tears showed their love.

Despite the healing power of tears, I sensed that the old woman was not at a place in her mourning to release them. For me to force her emotions would be to manipulate her own unique grieving process. Besides, her front had a protective purpose, which I later learned was to shield herself from the loss of yet another man in her life. "You've been here before . . ." I offered at one point. She closed her eyes tightly in a sort of painful confirmation.

"I can see it's important for you to be strong," I reflected as the old woman continued to pace the room. She nodded ardently and then sat down on the couch, disarming herself at least in part.

"If I'm not strong, then nobody else will be," she reasoned matter of factly.

"How about God?" I queried, inviting her to ponder the validity of her statement. She just sat still and silent, a marked contrast from her previous pacing and fidgeting, demanding and proclaiming. Her inactivity spoke louder than any words. I imagined a lightbulb flickering inside her head that was finally allowing her to take small steps toward trusting herself and the world around her.

Recognizing the urgency of Mr. Dixon's situation, I suggested that we pray for him. The three women agreed. "I just don't want Keith to suffer anymore," Mrs. Dixon pleaded in response to my question as to what I should be sure to include in prayer. "That God's will be done," Gina added. To my surprise, Mr. Dixon's mother simply affirmed the others' requests, as if she somehow had surrendered to the fact that God didn't need her directions.

After prayer, one of the nurses suddenly entered the room with an emergent message. "You better come now," she alerted. "His condition is quickly deteriorating." Apparently, God was answering our prayer in His own perfect way.

The three women and I made our way to Keith's room in a huddle of misery tempered by the knowledge of God's presence. After donning the protective garb used for patients in isolation, we surrounded Mr. Dixon at his bedside. His murky yellow eyes, jaundiced from liver failure, were still open. Mrs. Dixon took hold of her husband's emaciated and scaly hand, taking great comfort in the fact that he squeezed hers in return. Perhaps that was her dying husband's only way of expressing what he was so desperately trying to do: hold on. Treasuring what would be their last moment of connection, Mrs. Dixon smiled, licking tears into her mouth as they trickled down her cheeks. Suddenly, lightly touching his disintegrating nails, she let out an affectionate giggle. "Baby," she said, leaning over him in attempt to look into his eyes. "You better get well or I'm gonna have to give you a manicure!" We all laughed, appreciating the rare bittersweet moment that was drawing all too quickly toward extinction.

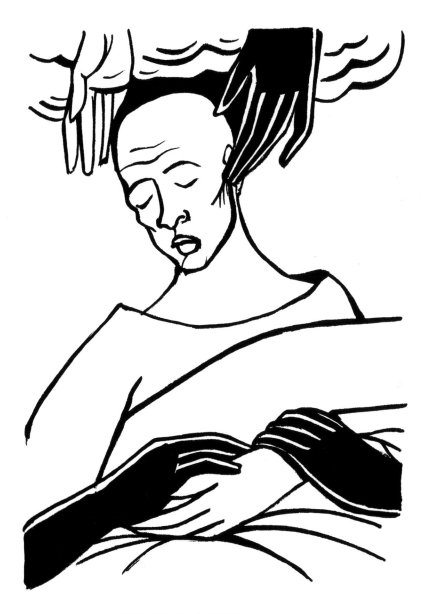

Glancing at the monitor, we noticed that Mr. Dixon's blood pressure was rapidly dropping, a trend that the nurse had been monitoring yet appeared hesitant to draw attention to. The worrisome reading of 70/50 from earlier that morning now seemed healthy compared the current one: a mere 35/28. Leaping to 150 beats per minute, his heart made one last final attempt to overcome his leaky vessels, only to eventually plunge.

Dr. Ulion entered the room, draping his arm around Mrs. Dixon. "We're going to turn off the monitor now, okay?" he offered. She slowly nodded in resignation. "I'm so sorry, Mrs. Dixon; I'm so sorry."

As the nurse was detaching the monitor, Gina suddenly fainted, collapsing against the wall in response to the intensity of the impending death. The horrible reality was too much for her senses to bear. Two nurses caught her and then carried her out to the corridor, placing smelling salts under her nose to revive her. They seemed to realize that she was the only one they could help. I glanced back and forth, from bedside to hallway, not knowing where to direct my attention.

My dilemma quickly solved itself, as Mr. Dixon, his wife, and I were suddenly left in the room behind a closed curtain. The medical team had graciously left us in the silence of the room to savor the sacred moment, a moment saturated with both tragedy and wonder, despair and hope, death and new life. As we stood in silent reverence, Mrs. Dixon slowly laid herself on her husband's chest, placing her hands on his head and cheek. And then she wept. With each moan of agony also came a sigh of relief, for with her beloved's life also went his suffering.

After several minutes, Mrs. Dixon lay still and silent on her husband's chest, as if she were sleeping. I wondered if, in a sense, she was at rest. Seemingly empty of tears, words, and emotions, seemingly empty of herself, she appeared ready and willing to be refilled, like a hungry child opening her hands for a cookie. Surrounded by such an essence of surrender and trust, she raised her body, rubbed her eyes, and gently smiled. "Well, he said he knew he was going to a better place. I want to call his people now," she whispered in a shaky voice, referring to Mr. Dixon's fellow Muslims. "I want to call them because that's what he wanted."

I smiled and nodded, my own teardrops making me all the more aware of the holy ground on which we walked. Holy ground—a place where grief in all its faces is welcome to be visited and revisited, transformed and retransformed into a stepping-stone toward God, whether we are conscious of it or not. In her desire to be strong, Mr. Dixon's mother came closer to her own weakness, the very place that gave way to God's power. In resuming his medical duties, Dr. Ulion found God's protection from the emotional toll of dealing with the death of yet another patient. In Gina's state of syncope, she encountered her own limits, inviting her to seek deeper communion with the God who knows no limits. In her act of surrendering her husband into God's hands, Mrs. Dixon enjoyed the peace that comes from entrusting our cares to our Maker. In his letting go of his life, Mr. Dixon himself fell into the open arms of God, returning to the very One to whom he belonged. And I, in partaking in the multiple mysteries of God's immanent presence, realized yet again that His light guides me wherever I am willing to follow.

—15—

Mutual Healing

"Oh, my butt hurts. It feels like it has barnacles in it," Mrs. Moore moaned. She was one-day postop, immobilized by her pain. The morphine didn't seem to be working. Part of me wanted to laugh out loud at Mrs. Moore's creative comment that seemed foreign coming out of this frail eighty-three-year-old woman's mouth, but I sensed that laughter and jokes were not what she needed now.

I knew from the moment I walked in Mrs. Moore's room that God had led me there. Her eyes said to me, "Please . . . just be with me. I'm hurting and I need someone. I need someone to listen and to care . . ."

After I introduced myself, her anxious posture seemed to relax as her head settled back into the pillow. Her mouth quivered, as if she was dying to let out a river of words that remained dammed up inside her head. "I'm so miserable," she finally said. I could tell that there were so many more words behind her thoughts, but that this was all she had the energy to express. Besides, the brief statement summed it all up.

I sat with Mrs. Moore in silence for several minutes. We were mere strangers in one sense, yet in another we seemed to feel at home as our eyes locked in a rare but comfortable gaze. I was hoping that she found the comfort in my eyes that I found in hers.

"Will you pray for me?" she asked. I accepted her invitation, wondering if I should have offered to do so earlier.

"Is there anything in particular on your mind that you want to pray about?" I asked. I cringed inside as I realized how dim-witted my question sounded. "My health, dummy," the insecure part of me envisioned her replying. But somehow I wanted to include her deepest concerns in prayer, concerns that I had not yet been able to discern.

"Just pray," she said simply. Perhaps she understood that God already knew her concerns and that I didn't need to, and that maybe she didn't even need to. Mrs. Moore's ease inspired me. She exuded a rare trust in the grace of God. "Maybe she should be the one leading our prayer," I thought to myself. I realized that, once again, God was using me, a ragamuffin of a servant, in the holiest of situations.

After our prayer, which I somehow managed to utter as I see-sawed between feelings of inadequacy and honor, Mrs. Moore kept her firm yet gentle grip on my hand. She stroked my hand, and then I began to wonder: "Who's comforting who here?" Our roles appeared to be temporarily reversed, yet I marveled at the notion that the moment was probably a healing one for her.

"I have two wonderful granddaughters," she sighed in a soft voice.

"Oh, really?" I felt privileged that she wanted to share some of her life with me.

"Yes," she replied. "Ten minutes apart." Mrs. Moore seemed to be partly in another world, reflecting on memories with her grand-daughters. I could see it in her eyes and hear it in her voice that she loved them very much. It seemed therapeutic for her to talk about them. I wondered if it was easing her pain. She was easing my pain, a pain I didn't even know I had. Aware of the transference that was going on, I felt like a beloved daughter, safe at her mother's breast. I felt at home, and I think Mrs. Moore did too.

Mrs. Moore drifted off to sleep. I awoke her slightly, letting her know that I was leaving so that she could rest. The nurse passed me on my way out. "Oh good, the morphine must be working," she said.

I just smiled and nodded. "Something like that," I thought to myself.

Free to Die

"Hello there, young lady," Mr. Newley greeted me in a fragile yet friendly tone, his voice possessing the gentleness of a pussy willow. As I walked into the old man's room, I felt as if I could be his granddaughter, coming to sit on Grandpa's lap for a bedtime story. In a sense, I was fulfilling this role, only I would not become completely aware of my privileged position until later that day.

As I introduced myself to Mr. Newley, I felt myself putting on the scanty armor of a professional chaplain. "Hello, Mr. Newley. My name is Chaplain TenBrook," I stated after clearing my voice and proceeding to lower it from its usual high pitch. I stood erect with my legs together and my arms crossed on my chest. Little did I know at that point that my body language was speaking louder than any formal introduction ever could, as if to say, "Yes, I *am* hiding something." Accustomed to comments in reference to my youthful looks, I was determined to get past the "You're too young to be a chaplain" remark. My defenses slowly started to dissolve, however, as Mr. Newley simply smiled at me and offered me a seat at his bedside.

"It's such a beautiful day," he said, peering around the curtain and out the window upon the cold, clear, and sunny November day.

"Yes, it is, isn't it?" I replied, feeling myself relax into the present moment.

"These kinds of fall days have always been my favorite," he began. "Ever since I was a child. I remember my brother and I used to build huge piles of leaves and then fall into them. Of course, Mother always wanted us to haul the leaves to the compost instead of making messes with them." He laughed as heartily as his weak lungs would allow, inviting me to look on with him at the picture of his past.

"That was a long time ago," he reflected with a nostalgic look in his eyes. "I'm the only one left now, here in Baltimore."

"Hmm, what's that like for you?" I asked, assuming that the suffocating loneliness I often feel in times of isolation would be his, as well.

"It's okay," he replied in a calm voice of resolution. "I know I'm not alone in here," he said, placing his swollen, needle-poked hand on his chest. Unlike me and so many, Mr. Newley seemed to possess an ability to find sufficient comfort within his memories. In this way, the old man appeared to enjoy intimate fellowship despite his solitary life.

"I have a granddaughter, and o-o-o-o she's a cutie!" he pronounced with a delightful chuckle. "She and her mommy live down in South Carolina. So precious, so precious, little Gaby. She calls me 'Gampy,' kind of a cross between grandpa and her own name." Mr. Newley beamed, and I sensed that his precious Gaby was very present in his heart. A few tears rolled down his cheeks, not tears of sadness, but rather tears of immense joy.

As I sat with Mr. Newley, it occurred to me that he didn't need the so-called professional mask I had initially brought with me. Rather, he needed a friend, a companion, a genuine person, perhaps even a granddaughter: someone who cared, someone who was willing to give him a receiving heart. In short, he needed *me*. None of my false selves to which I often resort would do. It then occurred to me that the me that Mr. Newley needed was also the me that I needed: the me that God made, high voice and all. Would I have the courage to simply let myself be shaped into the image of the One who formed and continues to form me?

Mr. Newley continued to share bits and pieces of his life with me: the way his wife, June, used to prepare a Thanksgiving feast as if the holiday was going out of style; the years he spent as a salesman going door to door, not because he liked the job but because he felt it was his duty to provide for his family; and how he was grieving the loss of his son who had recently succumbed to a long battle with cancer. The old man recounted his life in the fullness of all the emotions the events evoked: gladness and sadness, peace and pain, hope and despair. The only feeling he didn't appear to express was regret. He seemed to know that whatever had happened or hadn't happened, God's reconciling purpose transcended it all.

After spending thirty minutes or so together, Mr. Newley and I closed our time together in prayer. I cannot remember what we prayed about, only the feeling with which we prayed: peace. Perhaps our few words elude my memory because as we lifted them to God, I recall feeling as though He had already received and even answered them. As I write, I am reminded of Jesus' words with regard to prayer: ". . . your Father knows what you need before you ask him" (Matthew 6:8).

Mr. Newley and I embraced each other in a firm yet gentle hug, I leaning over his elevated bed. As I proceeded to make my way toward the door, we waved good-bye to each other, a benediction of sorts for whatever was to come. I felt truly full and blessed, my cup running over. I had found yet again that it was in my willingness to receive Mr. Newley that I had been able to partake in giving him what he needed.

I walked down to the cafeteria, as it was lunchtime. Having already been nourished, however, I found that I was not hungry for my usual bagel and frozen yogurt. All the same, I sat down at a table by the window, using my time there to savor and digest the delicious spiritual meal I had been granted.

About thirty minutes later, I headed back up to the Progressive Care Unit, wondering what God would have for me next. The blind woman with heart failure who loved to pray with whomever would hold her hand? The twenty-seven-year-old who was terrified to find himself with heart disease at such a young age? The old woman transferred from the psychiatric ward whose "irrational" fears of death were only intensified by the diagnosis of an underlying medical condition? No, none of these scenarios. In fact, any figment of my imagination could not prepare me for what I was about to discover.

As I walked down the hallway, I noticed a sign on Mr. Newley's door. "PLEASE SEE NURSE BEFORE ENTERING" it stated. I froze in my tracks in the middle of the corridor with a sense of foreboding, for such notices usually mean that the patient has gone into cardiac arrest or is in the midst of some emergent procedure. But Mr. Newley's room was still and quiet, lacking the frantic

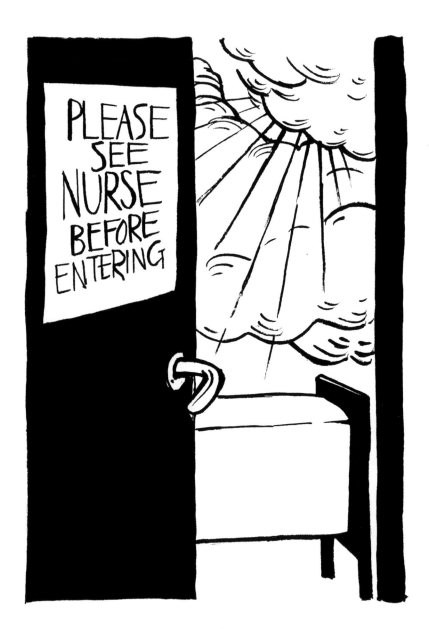

movements and urgent commands of doctors and nurses that usually characterize such situations. There was only one likely scenario left. "Could Mr. Newley have . . . have . . . ?"

In the midst of my fear-induced trance, Ned, the nurse, tapped my shoulder. I hesitated before turning my head, dreading what he would have to say to me. Deep down, I already knew. "Did he . . . ?" I began.

"Yes," Ned said, putting his hand on my shoulder.

As we both slowly made our way to the nurses' station, I found myself overcome by shock. "But I just saw him," I said to myself over and over again. "And he looked so well, so at peace, so full of life! He couldn't be dead!" Ned then explained that he had gone in to take Mr. Newley's vitals shortly after I had left, only to find him unresponsive, his body still warm yet limp and lifeless. They had not taken any action to revive him, as a DNR order had been in place.

I sat down in a chair in the corner of the station and rested my head on my hands in an attempt to digest the raw news that had come upon me when I least expected it. I wanted to regurgitate it and pretend it had never happened. Suddenly, one of the doctors who had cared for Mr. Newley poked me on the shoulder, interrupting my thoughts.

"So, that's the effect you have on people!" he howled, making an untimely attempt at a crude joke. I just looked up at him with a straight face, as if to say, "Come again?" He then darted back to his work, seemingly unable to take advantage of the opportunity to restore any sense of congeniality. Looking back, I wonder if the doctor was simply projecting his feelings of failure onto me, the only way he knew how to cope at that moment with his patient's death.

I then made my way back to Mr. Newley's room, taking advantage of the precious time to say good-bye, again. I sat down in the same chair that, like his hand, now felt cold and hard. "But I just saw him. He looked so well, so at peace, so full of life." These same words of confusion buzzed about my brain until they suddenly snapped as if their plugs had been pulled. They were then replaced by a clarity that settled on my heart and mind with the tenderness of a falling autumn leaf.

"But Gretchen," I said to myself, speaking from the voice of the One who wells up inside of me. "He *was* well, he *was* at peace, he *was* full of life. And it was precisely because of this that he was able to die." I sat in amazement of the blessed events in which I had partaken, realizing that in sharing his memories with me, Mr. Newley had been in the process of lifting his life back into the hands of the One who had first spoken it into being.

—17—

Light Shines in the Darkness

Mrs. Ingle thought that the devil had taken her over. The news of the referral from the psychiatric ward left me with a pit in my stomach, as I had never offered pastoral care to a patient with such a problem. "Oh, Lord, this is beyond me!" I said to myself and God at the same time. "I don't think I can handle this." I was right—the situation *was* beyond me and I *couldn't* handle it—but deep down, I sensed that it was for this very reason that God was calling me to respond to it. "Okay, Lord," I agreed with the One whose will would be done. "I'm going, and only because you're with me."

It didn't take me long to slip out of an open and obedient spirit. Temporarily consumed by fear of what to say to the seventy-three year-old Catholic woman, I made a detour to the conference room and began frantically looking up Bible verses that spoke of God's providence over evil. "Hmm," I thought to myself. "What scripture would help her?" As I anxiously flipped through my concordance, I asked the same question to Sue, one of the other chaplains.

"Why don't you just listen to her first?" she offered. Her simple yet profound statement served to remind me of my primary role, like a faithful tree marker on a dark and winding forest trail. Through her words, I learned that I need to look beyond myself for a balanced perspective instead of focusing only on the potholes I see in the path of my weary footsteps.

"What a novel idea!" I laughed, realizing how easily and frequently I get sidetracked by my own agenda. "Thank you, Sue!" My colleague had a knack for extending pastoral care not only to patients, but to anyone with whom God brought her in contact, including me!

I headed up to the ward as if a weight had been lifted from my shoulders, prompted by God, yet again, that it was His work to be done and not mine. I encounter this realization frequently, often in the form of humbling experiences that serve to remind me of my humanity. As much as I would like to think otherwise at times, I am not God, a recurrent revelation that can be disappointing or freeing depending upon how I receive it.

"ELOPEMENT RISK!" signs throughout the psychiatric ward seemed to scream at me as I made my way to the nurses' station. I have always hated those signs, for the high-tech words convey the exact message they seek to gloss over: "Don't let the crazy people get out!" I have often wondered if more hopeful and compassionate signs would diminish the fear that compels some patients to try to escape, such as "Healing Potential!" or "Make yourself at home. Love will soon be served." Unfortunately, I am not in a position to promote such environmental changes.

I introduced myself to Carol, the nurse who had called with the referral. "Mrs. Ingle thinks she's going to hell, and that there's nothing she can do about it," the soft-spoken woman said, her face grave with concern. "I don't know where she got the idea, but I was wondering if you could do something to dispel it."

"Well, I can offer her a place of comfort and encouragement in the midst of it," I responded, hoping not to disappoint the nurse that I knew of no quick solutions. "And perhaps in doing that, the idea will lose some of its power." In my experience, evil thoughts are best left subject to God's healing presence than to my attempts to explain them away. To dismiss Mrs. Ingle's fears would be to dismiss her reality, and ultimately to dismiss her.

I found Mrs. Ingle in the activity room sitting in a mobile chair. The petite woman's head barely peered over the tray table in front of her. She appeared to be looking out the window at the monotonous brick wall of the neighboring building, her expressionless face proclaiming the intensity of her mental anguish. I gently placed my hand on her shoulder and kneeled to make eye-level contact. I wanted to present myself as the equal that I am, for I did not know what I represented for her: God's judgment or His hope.

"Are you a Catholic priest?" she immediately asked expectantly in response to my introduction as "Chaplain TenBrook." Part of me wanted to laugh, for a twenty-six-year-old petite woman in a skirt and pumps is not frequently mistaken for a Catholic priest! But, bless her heart, Mrs. Ingle's innocent question deserved an answer that met her exactly where she was.

"No, I'm not," I replied in a soft voice, watching the hope disappear from her face like the sun during a lunar eclipse. Part of me wondered if I simply should have responded in the affirmative, conforming to whatever it was that the despondent woman thought she needed at the time. But then I reconsidered, realizing that I myself might end up on the psychiatric ward if I sought to minister to others under such a title. "But I can arrange for Father Phil to come up to see you if you like," I continued, in attempt to restore the little hope that she appeared to have.

"Yes, I would like that," she said. "Could he come up this afternoon?" Her question possessed an urgency that suggested a pain she could no longer bear.

"I'll try my best," I responded, having learned from past mistakes to never make promises with patients that you are not sure you can keep. "Is there anything *I* can do for you before then?"

"Well," she said hesitantly, as if unable to decide whether my ears could bear the weight of a deep and dark confession. "You see, I've sinned," she said, tears streaming down her face. Again, I admit that part of me wanted to laugh. "Welcome to the human race," I felt like saying. But, deep down I knew that such a reply would only serve to trivialize her pain.

"Is there something you think you have done to deserve punishment?" I queried, inviting her to release her burden.

"Oh, yes, I have sinned!" she exclaimed again. I remained silent, just letting her ambiguous confession rest in a safe place of acceptance. To force her to share any details would be to satisfy my curiosity, and to deny her the freedom to heal.

As I gazed upon Mrs. Ingle's frail body, collapsed onto the tray table, I was moved by her repentant spirit. I thought of Job, sitting in a pile of dust and despair, in a heap of ashes and agony, waiting patiently for the God he had come to know through—and only through—his suffering. Would Mrs. Ingle, too, be delivered from the depths of her darkness? At the same time, I was deeply saddened that Mrs. Ingle appeared unable to move on to the new life to which God was calling her. Her mind held her spirit hostage to a prison of some painful memory. How ironic it was that this woman who was so keenly aware of her need for forgiveness was unable to receive it.

"I just hope God forgives me," Mrs. Ingle whispered, lifting her head as if it weighed a ton. Her plea was not one of expectation, but of doubt.

"He already has," I whispered back, looking straight into her weary eyes. My words seemed to flow out naturally, the Truth inside of me longing to be proclaimed. Yet at the same time, I was uncertain as to whether or not they were helpful to her, for the words suggested that forgiveness was something that could be claimed on a whim. But it was not that easy for Mrs. Ingle, for even after several priests' pronouncements of absolution, she appeared unable to welcome God's grace into her heart. In fact, forgiveness seemed to elude her no matter how far she reached out for it. I hoped that one day she would have the courage to let it reach out to her.

After a few moments of silence, I asked Mrs. Ingle if she would like to close in prayer. "Yes, I guess to pray is all I can do now," she said with a sigh of resignation, as if prayer were a last resort versus a top priority. I have found myself operating from the same mind-set in the midst of my struggles, preferring any source of immediate comfort to the hopeful waiting to which prayer calls us. Ironically, it is from prayer itself that any lasting solace springs forth.

"What would you like to be sure to include in prayer?" I asked, hoping to minister to her needs and not my own.

"I need strength," she pleaded, "strength to decide if I'm just going to give in."

"Give in?" I reflected, sensing that this very idea that appeared pitiful on the surface was brimming with power at its core.

"Yes, to just let whatever happens happen." Her very words suggested a hope and a surrender of which she was not yet aware. Maybe Mrs. Ingle was unknowingly on the verge of letting God do what she could not: save herself.

After prayer, I offered Mrs. Ingle a hug. To my surprise, she immediately accepted the embrace, her characteristic fear and hesitancy seeming to dissolve in my arms. As we held each other, she whispered over and over again amid tears, "Forgive me, Lord. Forgive me, Lord. Forgive me, Lord." With each plea, her body seemed to grow more limp, as if to make way for the strength for which we had just prayed.

As I headed back downstairs, my heart welled up with joy, not because of what I had done, and not because of what Mrs. Ingle had done, but because of what God had done and would continue to do: bring His marvelous light into our darkness. "The light shines into the darkness, but the darkness has not understood it," says the Gospel of John (John 1:5). This verse comforts me, for it reminds me that wherever I go, God is with me. And because He is with me, the darkness that surrounds me has no choice but to succumb to His light, like a clump of dry sand when it is immersed in water. No, Mrs. Ingle did not escape her darkness, nor did I banish it from her, but together we had allowed it to become a dwelling place for the Light. And where there is Light, the darkness of evil cannot reign.

Good-bye, Grandmère

The thought of a baby had never come to mind when thinking about my grandmother. But that's exactly what popped into my head when I stood at her bedside on that late summer day at the nursing home. She lay curled up in a fetal position with the covers tucked firmly around her. Her freshly washed face appeared moist and rosy, yet expressionless, and her mouth quivered with occasional whimpers. "Yes, almost like a baby," I thought to myself. If it weren't for her sizable figure and mop of recently permed white hair, I might have thought I was in a nursery.

But I was not in a nursery, nor was I with a baby. I was with Grandmère, my maternal grandmother who has lived three times as many years as I have. Grandmère—that is what we have always called her, French for grandmother, although we never have adhered to the correct pronunciation. This hasn't seemed to matter, however, because the blatantly American way we say her name—"Gran' mare"—has served to set her apart, making her sound just as special as she always has been.

The Grandmère who lay in front of me on that day was not the Grandmère of my memories, however. Nor was she just another patient, like the countless other oldsters I have visited in hospital ministry. No, our roots were too deep for any sense of objectivity. In fact, they were so deeply entwined in the soil of our lives that I felt threatened by the fragile state of her withering condition. I longed for the *real* Grandmère: the one who took me to Arch Cape for weekends at the beach; the one who ironed my grandfather's shirts while watching *One Life to Live* and sipping her afternoon cup of Kava; the one who fed the crusts of her morning toast to Smuckers, the faithful black Lab; the one who baked what seemed a thousand tins of Norwegian lefse for family and friends at Christmastime. But the Grandmère I knew was gone, ransacked by a thief called Alzheimer's disease. The dreaded diagnosis had progressed quickly, leaving her mind a prisoner to her body, a body that until recently had functioned as if it were twenty years younger. But now, the disease process was infesting her entire being. Her speech consisted of mere gibberish. Her arms and legs shook in brief and regular pulses—"ministrokes" the doctor had said. She wore diapers, too. Yes, almost like a baby.

I don't visit my grandmother very often, about once every couple of years, as she and I live on opposite coasts. Each time I see her, I am amazed by how her condition has deteriorated. It started back when I was in high school when one day she phoned in tears. Lost downtown with an armful of shopping bags, she was unable to remember where she had parked the old silver Volvo. I remember how terrified she was, not about losing the car, but about what the incident suggested about her. She mentioned nothing of this, but her unbridled tears and fidgeting fingers said it all: she dreaded what was to come and feared the inevitable conclusion.

The phone calls became more frequent, yet their pleas for help progressed from mere statements of fear to those of anger. "Why did you leave without telling me?!" she would shriek in the midst of a hallucination. "But, Grandmère, we were never there . . ." I would begin, only to hear the line click at the other end. Grandmère was not interested in answers that didn't make sense to her, in answers that only served to confirm the dementia she so deeply feared. To scream and yell in outrage, to blame everyone and everything around her: this was the only control she had on her world, a world she could no longer trust.

After Grandmère regularly began leaving the stove on and climbing into bed at ten o'clock in the morning, my family decided it was time to move her to an assisted living center. Such an institution is supposed to be a less threatening name for a nursing home, a community whose residents require less intensive medical care. But whatever it was called, Grandmère experienced it as another assault on her independence, further proof that she really was "going crazy," a scenario she often bitterly proposed.

The moving day is vivid in my memory. With my parents gently leading her arm-in-arm into the facility, she was initially quite content and, in fact, intrigued with the lovely building and its pristine surrounding landscape. However, when she saw her name written on an apartment door and realized she was to live there, her serenity turned to protest. She broke her arms loose and threw her purse violently across the room. Several other residents sitting in the living room stared listlessly at her. Perhaps they had all been in that place before, too. Soon Grandmère would react to her new neighbors in the same way.

Now, as I stood at Grandmère's bedside years later, all of these memories flooded my mind like a tidal wave, a sharp contrast to the stillness of her present state. Lying motionless on the bed, seemingly void of any thought or emotion, she reminded me of a frozen computer screen indefinitely stuck in a state of nothingness. Given the poor likelihood that she would ever spontaneously reboot, would it not be better if she just shut down? This question left me with a sense of guilt that gnawed at me like a bleeding ulcer. "Do I really want my own grandmother to die?" I remember thinking to myself. In many ways, it seemed as though she already had.

In an attempt to make a connection—any connection—with Grandmère, I caressed her hand hoping it would awaken her from her slumber. Her eyes slowly cracked open and she turned her face up from the pillow, looking right through me and gently giggling. I wondered what she saw. Did I look funny, was God telling her jokes, or was she just experiencing another dying synapse? I wanted to make eye contact with her. It seemed this was the only means of genuine relationship left; exchanging words of love and care or embracing in an intimate hug were no longer options.

"Hi, Grandmère," I uttered in a soft yet cheerful voice, kneeling at her bedside and smiling into her vacant eyes. "Remember me? I'm Gretchen, Terry's daughter." I knew my words made little sense to her, but I hoped that the tender way in which I tried to offer them would provide a loving message that even she could understand.

Apparently, she did understand the message. To my delight, she gazed directly into my eyes and whispered, "Oh, yes." Beaming with truly unspeakable joy, she appeared to be savoring the rare moment of togetherness that her disjointed world almost never allowed. Yes, the real Grandmère was back, even if only briefly.

The precious moment came and went quickly, lasting no more than ten seconds. Before I could respond to her, she was looking beyond me again, laughing at what appeared to be nothing in particular. I felt as if I had walked over a heat vent on a cold city street, and I wanted to go back to that warm place forever. But then I realized that if such a plea were granted me, Grandmère's gift of genuine connection would no longer hold the cherished place in my heart that it now does. Like a delicate flower in the open palm of my hand, it was meant to be received and adored, not crushed and distorted.

As my family and I left the nursing home that day, I wept, not knowing whether I was feeling bittersweet joy or profound sadness. On the one hand, I was struck by the fact that in Grandmère's most helpless and dependent state, she had gifted me with a blessed treasure: a moment of genuine love and connection that even a gold-medal Olympic athlete could not offer. At the same time, I was angry that Grandmère had been cheated of so many other opportunities to experience such communion with others. Like a fish out of water, she was left to suffocate indefinitely, sustained only by an occasional splash. But then it occurred to me that perhaps if she were saturated with endless possibilities to reach out to others, she would be just another typical adult, blindly wading through the mystery of life. Yes, just like me and so many others, she might forfeit the privilege of love, failing to nourish her own and others' hearts with the sustenance of a God who waits patiently to provide.

I sense that I will never truly see Grandmère again in this world. In that respect, the momentary bond with which we were blessed was as much of a greeting as it was a farewell, as much of a hello as it was a good-bye. The next time I see her, if there is a next time, the Alzheimer's will likely have taken another bite out of her being, leaving the landscape of her life even more barren than it already is. Receding further into infancy, she will have become more and more like a baby. Yes, more and more like a baby. But instead of growing in her interaction with and attachment to the world, she would finally be set free from it.

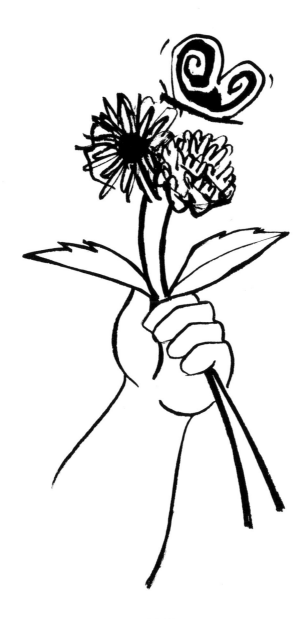

—19—

Addicted to Pain

Ms. Daniels held the white sheet taut under her chin, like a child afraid of ghosts under the bed. Her room was still and dark: the shades drawn, the lights out, and the TV off. If it weren't for the form of her body under the sheet, I might have thought that the room was empty. And it if weren't for her bug-eyed gaze over the sheet, I might have thought that she was dead. Even though Ms. Daniels was indeed alive, her room greeted me with a helpless sense of sterility.

The twenty-one-year-old was enduring her second day in the hospital, admitted because of an infected ulcer on her foot due to IV drug abuse. I happened upon her while making rounds on the ward. "Hi," she said listlessly after I introduced myself, her voice barely making its way across the room.

"How are you feeling today?" I asked, trying to get a sense of her receptivity to my visit.

"I'm okay; just tired I guess," she muttered, letting her head roll to one side of the pillow. Her lifeless words suggested an overall apathy about her situation.

"Would you like me to let you rest for now?" I asked, still uncertain as to whether or not she wanted me present.

"Oh, no, that's okay," she quickly responded, like a thready pulse that was finally giving way to a palpable beat. She pointed to the chair at her bedside.

"My foot . . . they had to cut part of it off," she stated matter of factly, pointing to the bump under the sheet at the end of the bed. I just nodded in response, my wrinkled forehead and pursed lips conveying my concern.

"Yeah, if I had waited any longer, they say they would have had to cut the *whole thing* off," she remarked, shaking her head in a way that suggested both disbelief and shame. "But they say I get to go home soon." Her words continued to float through the air with the force of a lazy summer breeze.

"You must be looking forward to going home," I offered, falling into the trap of assumptions. The comment had seemed like an easy way out, as I didn't know quite what to say about her foot surgery, knowing that the problem was drug related.

"Well actually, I'm not really looking forward to going home," she corrected me. "You know, I'm just going to *use* again." Ms. Daniels appeared to be more comfortable with the prospect of sharing her drug addiction than I was. Her openness surprised me initially, as often patients with addictions try their best to hide their problems to escape detection, confrontation, and the inevitable call for abstinence. But somehow, in her brief yet lethargic manner, Ms. Daniels made herself vulnerable to me in sharing the details of her broken life. Perhaps she felt she had nothing left to lose, and as I would soon learn, no one else to turn to.

"There's just no way I can stop using," she continued in an indifferent tone. "Drugs are everywhere, and I don't have nowhere to go. My godaunt—I live with her—she uses, too. My father, he already killed himself through drugs. My mother, she kicked me out and won't even let me see my son. My boyfriend, he just up and left. And my grandfather, he refuses to see me since I been taking his money." Ms. Daniels just stared at the ceiling in a state of hopelessness. Normally, such a string of misfortunes would provoke tears, yet the young woman seemed void of any emotions, as if they too were no longer available to her.

Listening to Ms. Daniels, I wondered what had led her to drugs in the first place. Perhaps she had learned of them from her godaunt after having been forced out of her mother's house, pregnant and unwed. Maybe she had simply followed in her father's footsteps, and now feared for her own survival. In any case, her life had to be so painful that she resorted to the deceptive refuge of drugs, only to cause herself more pain in the long run. Ironically, in trying to run away from her pain, she was bringing even more of it upon herself. In this way, Ms. Daniels was not only addicted to the ever-shrinking escape that drugs allowed her, but also to the ever-growing pain they caused her. Would she let her pain destroy her or would she finally listen to the message it was trying to send her? The very pain that was ruining her was also trying to save her.

Pain, the sensation we go to great lengths to avoid, presents a certain paradox. Like a faithful watchman, it calls out to warn us of impending danger. At first, it calls out softly, perhaps in the form of a bleeding scratch, a teardrop, or a heartache. But then, when we ignore it, it speaks louder to get our attention, until it finally resorts to violent screams. The unplanned pregnancy, the loss of her father, getting kicked out of her mother's house—perhaps these events had all served as mini-sirens alerting to the hurts in her heart that needed Love's healing. But when Ms. Daniels was unwilling to heed the warning, it came again in the guise of heroin overdoses, damaged relationships, and alienation. Now, it came in the form of a foot that needed to be partially amputated. How would Ms. Daniels' cry for help manifest itself next? Would she be willing to listen to it before it killed her?

Suddenly, the IV pump started to beep, sending its obnoxious signal throughout the room. "Oh, shut up," Ms. Daniels moaned, tapping the "Alarm Silence" button on the display. Interestingly, I noticed that she ignored the warning from her IV pump in the same way that she did any threat in her life.

"I can go get the nurse," I offered.

"No, that's okay. It always does this," she replied. Her statement echoed loudly inside my mind: "It always does this . . ." Ms. Daniels' life was in many ways a perpetual reaction, or lack thereof, to this very observation. The pain would keep coming, and she would keep ignoring it, only to find some other self-destructive behavior that brought her temporary relief. How I wished she could see the vicious cycle in which she was imprisoning herself. Little did she know that God was right there with her in her misery, appealing to her through one of His most powerful communicators —pain.

As I reflected on Ms. Daniels' situation, however, I was humbled to realize that I, too, have my own addiction. No, it is not drugs, but rather busyness, my deceptive source of calm that often serves to deter me from the very place I need to be: alone with God. In other words, consumed with fear that God will reveal something to me that I don't want to contend with, I often seek out other people or things to keep me busy so that I won't have to listen for His voice.

Consequently, I resort to taking up others' time unnecessarily, embarking on errands or chores that really don't need to be done, and ultimately, denying myself the genuine fulfillment of desires that only God, not people or things, can offer me. Like Ms. Daniels, I have a daily decision to make: will I run from the One who calls to me through my painful longings, or will I flee from Him to my own futile resources? Yes, pain can be our friend or our enemy. And like lepers who are unable to sense pain, we can habitually become unaware of our pain, digging ourselves deeper and deeper into a bottomless pit.

"I'm concerned about you," I said in the silence of the stilled alarm, offering with my comment yet another warning signal to replace that of the IV pump. Ms. Daniels just looked at me, listening to my words but appearing not to hear them.

"Well, that's nice and all," she replied. "But I just don't think I'm going to be able to stop." My heart sank when she said this. I longed to help her, but then realized that she would first need to be willing to help herself. I could only offer her a safe place to make that choice.

"Can you let children into the hospital?" she suddenly asked, changing the subject to yet again avoid more pain.

"It depends on the age," I responded, trying my best not to encourage the diversion.

"Well, I want to bring my son in," she said, smiling at the thought of him. "That will make me feel better." And yes, it probably would, but only on the surface. Then the original pain from which she had been running her whole life would resurface, screaming like a baby waiting to be embraced and fed. What would she use to cover it up next? Probably more pain, disguised in clothes of comfort.

My visit with Ms. Daniels ended on a dismal note. In expressing my concern for her, I threatened the life of the very thing that was killing her: drugs. She distanced herself from me, changing our conversation to what seemed to be the only subject left that could serve as anesthesia: her son. I found myself, yet again, in the place of powerlessness. Since then I have wondered if God, even in the midst of His power, at times feels powerless, for He continuously offers to us eternal healing, only to be rejected as we flee to worldly remedies. Addicted to the pain that we bring upon ourselves, we run from the very One whose desire is to speak to us through it.

—20—

A Time for Everything

The call to the Pediatric ICU came at a time when I felt I had absolutely nothing to offer. Overwhelmed with my own problems, I had resigned to leaving early that day. Just as I was putting on my coat and digging for my car keys, my beeper buzzed. "There's a one-year-old in the PICU who's going downhill pretty quickly," Margaret, the secretary, relayed the urgent message. I stood helplessly next to her desk, like a child who had been called to the principal's office. Staring at the floor and taking a deep breath, I let my bag drop with a kerplunk.

"I just don't think I can do this today, Margaret," I said, scanning the yellow referral card in my hand. Sensing my weariness, the kind and gentle woman made her way around the desk and offered me her open arms of love. I fell into them and sobbed, finding in her a safe place to "let it all out" without the need for words. Margaret seemed to appreciate that it was not the details of my suffering that needed to be lifted to God, but only the hurt behind them. Little does Margaret know, even to this day, that with her loving spirit she often serves as the chaplain to the chaplaincy department.

Eventually depleted of my own tears, I felt cleansed and renewed by those of God, the God who walks with me through my valleys as well as over my peaks. Somehow, in my inability to be strong, I sensed God's strength; in my limited capacities, I felt God's abundant provision. Even though I witness daily God's transforming power in the lives of others, somehow I am still always surprised when it befalls me.

"I think I can do this, Margaret," I finally said, looking at the opportunity for service in a new light. Yet again, I was reminded that my ministry was not my ministry, but God's, and that anything

I had to offer would not be mine, but God's. Stripped of my mask of self-sufficiency, I had no choice but to let God do in me what only He could do: offer comfort to His people. Just as there had been a time for me to bewail my own bewilderment with Margaret, I sensed that now there was a time for me to put it aside to enter another's.

The PICU was a typical flurry of activity: doctors, nurses, and social workers scurrying up and down its halls; distraught family members seeking impossible refuge in the waiting room; beeping and wheezing machines keeping children "alive" in spite of their lifeless states; occasional reassuring cries from the mouths of terrified babes. Directed by the unit secretary, I made my way to the conference room, where the Morrison family was awaiting an update from Dr. Gray on little David's deteriorating condition. The toddler's life had been hanging on the thread of the ECMO (Extra Corporeal Membrane Oxygenation) machine, a new technology used to support both heart and lung function in gravely ill patients. But to everyone's horror, David had suffered the rare risk of bleeding to the brain as a result of the anticoagulants used to thin his artificially pumped blood. The devastating hemorrhage had left the little one brain dead. It appeared that just as there had been a time for David to live, there now was a time for him to die.

I knocked gently on the conference room door and entered, immediately taken aback by the number of mourning family members present: nine. They sat in heaps of despair, some sharing chairs, some sitting on the floor. As I introduced myself, they all looked up at me, seemingly too exhausted to acknowledge my presence with words. "Lord, help me! Where do I start?" I said to myself, gazing upon the flock of family members and knowing that each one was at a unique place in the course of grieving. Grief is a highly individual process driven by the culmination of all that one has been, is, and expects to be; it is a process over which the mourner has no control and over which I have no control. In the midst of my insecurity, however, I remembered that I was not responsible for each and every person's thoughts and emotions, but was simply called to be present with them in whatever they were experiencing, just as they were present to one another.

Dr. Gray entered the crowded room, followed by a string of nurses and the social worker. As we stuffed ourselves into the little room, I felt like a sardine and wondered if my presence was a help or a hindrance. It then occurred to me that I had forgotten to verify the source of the referral: the staff or the family? Such information is helpful, as some families understandably feel intruded upon when a chaplain is called without their knowledge. In any case, I knew that we *all* needed pastoral care, whether we recognized it or not. And the pastoral care could find its expression in a multitude of ways: from the sharing of hurt and anger, to prayer, to the holding of hands, and even to the willingness on my part to accept that the situation was not mine to handle. Time and time again, I realize that pastoral care is a discipline of discernment, a sensitivity to the Spirit's leading in the sacrament of the present moment. In pastoral care, there is a time for everything.

"I'm afraid I don't have any good news for you," Dr. Gray began with a solemn look on his face. "It looks like David has suffered a significant bleed to the brain . . ." Before the pediatric intensivist had a chance to continue, Mrs. Morrison slid from her chair to the floor, screamed, and began to pound the edge of the tabletop in front of her. "Oh, God, no!" she yelled repeatedly. The rest of the family buried their heads in their hands and joined in the earsplitting exhibition of anguish, seeming to know that Mrs. Morrison did not need their restraint but rather their fellowship in her grief. It was a time for rage.

As I pushed the table toward the corner to protect Mrs. Morrison from injuring herself, one of the nurses fetched some pillows for the same purpose. Scrambling on the floor like a mouse caught in a trap and punching the pillows with forceful blows, Mrs. Morrison reminded me of Jacob wrestling with God (Genesis 32:22-32). Just as Jacob would not cease his struggling with God until He blessed him, Mrs. Morrison would not withhold her rage until she was able to find a place of rest at its core. In her courageous persistence to "duke it out" with the Divine, God's healing would begin to flow freely like blood from an eternal wound.

Suddenly, Mrs. Morrison's mother stood up over her daughter, raised her arms in a gesture of supplication, and began to pray. "Oh, Lord Jeeesus! We beseech thee, Lord Jeeesus!" she proclaimed at the top of her lungs, the rest of the family affirming her words with additional "Yes, Lord Jeeesuses!" It seemed as though the meeting in the conference room had been temporarily transferred into a Pentecostal revival. The doctor and nurses stared at me, as though they expected me to restore order to the courtroom of sorts. I just closed my eyes and joined in the prayer, recognizing that the family was exactly where it needed to be: in the grasp of the Great Physician, in the hands of the Healer of the human condition.

After Mrs. Morrison and her family had calmed down, Dr. Gray resumed his brief yet precise explanation of David's tragic situation. Because the toddler no longer possessed any detectable brain function, it was now only a matter of time before Mr. and Mrs. Morrison would decide to remove their child from life support. To remove a loved one from life support is an agonizing decision that often leaves its makers forever oscillating between poles of horrifying guilt and despondent relief. Even though David had already died in a sense, the "pulling of the plug" would serve as the final wrecking ball to an already abandoned and ransacked city row house. The other children in the neighborhood had hope for renovation. But David's house was to be carried away, its only hope grounded in the fact that something new and beautiful would be resurrected in its place. To face this reality would be excruciatingly painful for the little boy's parents, but necessary all the same.

"I just . . . don't want him . . . to suffer," Mr. Morrison blurted between sobs in response to Dr. Gray's assertion that David's life was no longer salvageable. "I think . . . we need to take him . . . off that machine . . . and let him go home." Mrs. Morrision nodded in silent affirmation, as the rest of the family followed with several "Amens!" and "Take him, Lord Jeeesuses!" I was surprised initially by the consensus among the group, as it often takes different mourners different amounts of time to let go of their loved ones, for they are not only to lose those persons, but also parts of themselves.. At the same time, I realized that the family had been all along a unified force of strength, allowing their multitude of thoughts and emotions to drive them together through the pain, rather than succumbing to their destructive power to divide. Just as there had been a time for protest, there was also now a time for acceptance.

Suddenly, Mr. Morrison leaned over between his legs and threw up. Apparently, the dreadful reality was too much to handle at the moment. Like an overstuffed turkey, the man needed to unload some of his misery so he could accommodate what had already been packed inside of him. As the vomit splattered on the floor, I quickly handed the grieving father a dish in which to spit, and placed paper towels over the sour-smelling mess. The rest of the family barely reacted to Mr. Morrison's illness, probably because it seemed insignificant compared to the one before them that knew no cure.

After confirming Mr. and Mrs. Morrison's decision to remove David from life support, Dr. Gray asked them if they would like to hold the child while this was done. "Oh, yes, I want to be with my baby!" Mrs. Morrison cried immediately. Mr. Morrison agreed, and the two followed Dr. Gray into the hallway.

As the medical team prepared to extract the numerous tubes projecting from David's body, the family stood helplessly in the hallway, watching the events of the real-life nightmare unfold before their very eyes. Mrs. Morrison leaned against the wall across from David's room, her head cocked as she stared at the ceiling. Sensing her agony, I stood next to her and gently stroked her shoulder. She remained motionless for a moment, and then suddenly planted her soggy box of tissues in my hand and walked down the hallway toward the conference room. My first inclination was to take her rejection of sorts personally, but I held my narcissism in check, realizing that the mother's actions were not about me, but rather about the situation at hand. Mrs. Morrison was not rejecting me; she was rejecting the senseless loss of her only child. Looking back on that poignant moment, I realize that while pastoral care often involves the ministry of touch, a powerful medium of God's healing presence in one another, it also can involve the ministry of not touching, a critical means for conveying respect to those who seek to find rest in God, and in God alone. Yes, there is a time to embrace and a time to refrain from embracing.

Mrs. Morrison sat in a rocking chair in David's room, the lifeless child wrapped in a blanket on her lap. With her husband beside her, the two leaned over their little boy and wept fiercely, their cries audible throughout the entire unit. It was a time for weeping and

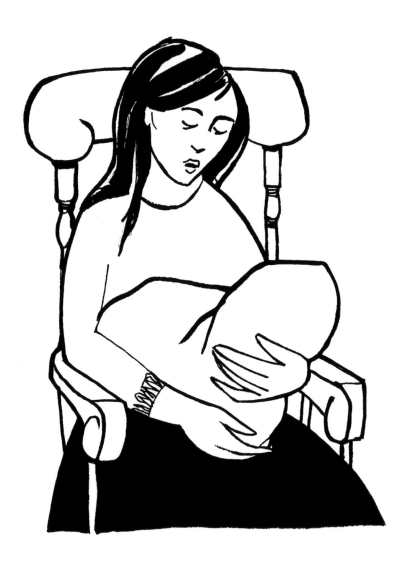

mourning, for the blessed gift that together they had received from the hands of God was now the beloved creation that together they would give back.

Part of me longed to enter the dark room where the threesome was spending its final precious moments together. But deep down, I knew that this was their time, and their time alone. To intrude would be to interfere, to seek a false comfort in a time that was not meant to be comfortable, to rob the moment of its painfully productive purity.

As I headed toward the elevator, I realized that during my time with the Morrison family, I had spoken not one word. Such visits are exceedingly rare, for I usually find silence difficult. Longing to transform a painful experience into something more palatable, I often blurt out empty words that only serve to distort the sacred nature of the present reality. However, with the Morrison family, God's call for silence and surrender had been so strong that my mouth knew no words to utter. It had been a time for silence as opposed to a time for speaking.

Looking back on that day so pregnant with ripe emotions, I recognize that there is truly a time for everything, despite whether the time and event be according to our self-centered schedules. Whatever a day brings with it, joy or sorrow, peace or pain, God's transcendent power meets us in our vast array of human experiences. As it is written, "There is a time for everything, and a season for every activity under heaven" (Ecclesiastes 3:1).

21

God's Poster Child

Ruth was by far the youngest patient in the Cardiac Care Unit. The twenty-year-old-Native American sat propped up in her elevated bed, hiding behind the bedside table that hung over her lap. She was cordial, having welcomed my unplanned visit with a smile and a handshake. In fact, she had seemed more concerned about my comfort than hers. Yet, at the same time, she appeared anxious and agitated, ripping the ball of tissues in her hands into tiny shreds.

"I just have these emotional times," she responded to my initial question about how she was feeling that day. I sensed that there was a river of feelings behind her words, waiting to flow from her with the urgency of mountain run-off after a long snowy winter.

"Hmm, what's that like?" I asked, offering her a place to unload. She immediately burst into tears, her hands clenching her knees with each sob like two powerful wrenches.

"Oh, I shouldn't pity myself!" she resigned, contorting her face into a rigid grimace and shaking her head back and forth as if it were a windshield wiper fighting a fierce rainstorm. Her fervent distress suggested underlying anger to me, a potentially productive or destructive emotion, depending upon how it is expressed. I sensed that I needed to allow her a place to release her anger, for it was bubbling like hot lava in a brewing volcano. After what I sensed had been confinement to a state of dormancy, she was ready to erupt.

"You don't think you should pity yourself . . ." I reflected, again inviting her to expand on the feelings hiding behind her few words.

"Yeah. You know, I could have died the other day when I went into arrest, but God saved me." Her words began spewing forth with the intensity of bullets from a machine gun. "In fact, he's saved me three times in my life. You see, I've been sick since I was born. I've had seizures all of my life. And just when I was starting to get strong, I got this—this heart problem they say they can't fix. They say that God doesn't give you more than you can handle. But this—this is more than I can handle!" She clenched her fists and pounded them on the tray table in front of her, causing a beverage cup on her barely touched breakfast tray to spout orange juice into the air, adding to the mess of her life.

"It sounds like you feel pretty helpless," I echoed. She nodded vigorously. As I stroked her hot and sweaty back, I imagined her blood literally boiling inside her. If she did not find an outlet to vent steam, the pressure would kill her. Perhaps it already was killing her. At the same time, I knew that while her anger could harm her, it could also save her. "Listen to me, Ruth!" it reverberated throughout her panicky body. "I need you to listen or else I will destroy you!" Perhaps Ruth was finally giving her anger a voice.

Ruth had every reason to be angry, for her life had been one tragedy after another. She was plagued by lifelong epilepsy and now by a recently diagnosed cardiomyopathy. And, as she would confide to me in a later visit, she had been raped at the age of fifteen by her cousin, now dead after a drug-related shooting. Her parents had demanded that she not tell anyone about the event, seeking to cover it up as if it had never happened, as if it were their daughter's own fault. It appeared that Ruth's life was grounded in suffering, a suffering that she could display but not explain, expose but not explore.

"I just don't know why all this is happening to me!" she protested, scratching the surface of the years of past hurts. "My mom tries to make me feel better by telling me that God is using me to show others how to have faith through trials. But I don't want to be some poster child!" Poster child—the title evoked powerful images of suffering in my mind, like that of a naked Ethiopian boy, his belly bloated from starvation and his face dotted with flies that he no longer had the energy to swipe away. Looking at such a picture, I am made to realize how fortunate I am. But at whose expense? At the little Ethiopian boy's, at the homeless person's, at the defenseless quadriplegic's? At Ruth's expense? Often the pain of being human does not seem worth the price.

"Maybe God wants me to die now so that everyone will marvel at how I've suffered!" she yelled, mocking the untimely perspective that I imagined had been preached at her more than once. I sensed that Ruth had been offered countless opportunities at martyrdom, but very few at personhood. While others freely sucked gratitude for their own lives from hers, few would receive the humanity that her hidden heart longed to share.

"I'm not ready to die yet!" she continued in a fit of healthy rage. Dependent on a heart transplant for long-term survival, Ruth was facing death eye to eye when she had not yet even had the chance to live.

"What is it that scares you about death the most?" I probed, hoping to continue to give her the rare opportunity to share her deepest fears.

"It's not the dying part," she explained in a quivering voice. "It's what I will leave behind . . . or actually what I *won't* leave behind. You see, I want to have a child myself. I want to give the man I love a part of myself. But they say I won't be able to have kids, but it's all I want, it's all I want . . ." She burst into a tirade of grief-stricken tears. Even though Ruth had not died, she was already grieving the life she had not, and would not, be able to live.

"I just want to have a child and watch it grow," she pleaded, looking somewhere beyond the ceiling and lifting her shaking hands into the air. "I want to watch it have all its firsts!" I could see that while the thought was a painful one, to share it eased her suffering. I wondered if anyone had ever asked her about her dreams before, if anyone had ever sought to nurture Ruth herself instead of the suffering that she had been hiding behind over the years.

"It seems that you want to have a child to experience the life that you can't, or never could have," I offered, recognizing that her hopes and dreams were not confined to herself.

"Yeah, I don't even remember my childhood," she said, shaking her head in disgust. "I was born to be sick!" Born to be sick . . .

In the midst of her telling statement, the phone suddenly rang. Ruth picked it up immediately with a sigh, probably more out of obligation than a desire to talk.

"Hi, Mom . . . I'm talking to the chaplain . . . She's just listening to me . . . I'll tell you later." She hung up the phone, falling into yet another well of tears.

"I made my mom upset," she stated in the form of a confession. "I always make her upset!"

"You *make* her upset?" I clarified. Somehow, Ruth had assumed responsibility for her mother's feelings, an unbearable burden for anyone. Apparently, Ruth's mother was allowed to get upset in the presence of her daughter, but Ruth herself was not granted such a privilege. Like many young women I see, including myself, Ruth was attempting to save others from their suffering at the expense of losing herself in the very process.

"Oh, I'm so sorry to dump all this on you!" she confessed yet again, eluding my question that, if received, had the power to set her free. Instead, she reverted to the torture of her own secure cage, seeming to think she was liable for my feelings as well.

Our momentous conversation was brought to a sudden halt with the abrupt entrance of the nurse. She planted a pile of ten or more pills and a cup of water in Ruth's hands, then stood erect with her arms crossed to watch the trembling young woman ingest them. "What's wrong?" the nurse queried in a whiny voice, as if any sign of upset were not allowed after surviving a heart attack. "I hope you feel better," she said, oblivious to Ruth's response that she was having a hard day, and then scurried out the door.

"How did that nurse make you feel?" I asked Ruth, wondering if her desire to take care of others would finally give way to her underlying anger of never being cared for herself.

"She doesn't like people to be upset," she responded in a simple tone, as if she had seen the scenario over and over again. Ruth was right: the nurse and countless others didn't like to see her upset. What Ruth failed to recognize, however, was that their desires, although sincere, were most likely based on *their* needs to feel okay about themselves, and not on an awareness of *her* needs. This is a pattern I see often in the context of pastoral care, and in relationships in general, for it is easier to express heartfelt wishes or attempt to solve sufferers' problems than it is to accompany them on their journeys of pain. In the former, we can assert a certain degree of control over others' problems and walk away from them in our own timing, at least temporarily. This makes us feel as if we have helped in some measurable way. But when we choose to befriend sufferers, we, too, become powerless and experience the vulnerability that we normally hide with our health, talents, and abilities. Ironically, it is often through this process that we find our true strength—the strength that is greater than ourselves and all things, the strength that only God can provide. Furthermore, the sufferer usually finds strength in no longer being alone, but unified in a powerlessness that gives way to peace.

As I sat with Ruth, I hoped that all who cared for her, including myself, would be willing to walk with her on the present path of pain instead of simply directing her to our own destinations or reminding her of where we would like her to finally arrive. With this in mind, I continued to accompany Ruth in her flurry of exploding emotion.

"Maybe you need to be upset," I offered, again trying my best to provide an outlet for her anger—anger that appeared to be discouraged in the company of many others.

"Yes, I do!" she suddenly proclaimed after digesting my comment. "People just want me to be happy and chipper all the time, but I'm not! My grandfather was that way right before he died, and look what it got him!" She continued to cry, both moaning in helplessness and screaming in rage.

"So if you express hope and happiness, you fear your own dying, and if you express doubt and anger, then you fear for everyone else," I reflected. Suddenly it occurred to me that Ruth had placed herself in an impossible situation. Like a timid child in a dark corner wearing a clown's mask, she oscillated between futile attempts to save herself and others. I could see that she was getting weary of playing this game that could only be lost, and never won.

"I just want to . . . live," she finally whispered in a strengthening surrender after several minutes of silence. As I embraced her ravaged body, I felt her boiling anger starting to convert itself into the reassuring steam I had envisioned earlier. At the same time, I sensed her ashes of despair beginning to transform themselves into stepping-stones of hope in the promise of restoration.

"I think you have just started to live," I offered. Ruth smiled at me and continued to cry, her tears of divine release turning my blouse into a sacred garment.

22

A Longing for Companionship

"Somebody get me a drink of water!" I heard a scraggly voice yell from the room at the west end of the ortho-trauma ward. The nurses just looked at each other and rolled their eyes. "Not Mr. Gregory again!" one of them groaned. The eighty-three-year-old man who was recovering from a hip replacement had been "driving them crazy" all morning long with his endless demands: more pain medication, the TV clicker he couldn't find, some tissues, to be moved to his bed and then back to the chair again, and, now, a drink of water. As I listened to Mr. Gregory's angry yet helpless cries, I sensed that it was not just the water he wanted, but the company of the person who would finally bring it to him. Unfortunately, the nurses did not have this luxury, so I took advantage of the opportunity to offer myself to him as a friend.

With a cup of ice water in my hand, I knocked on the open door and peered around the corner. I was greeted by Mr. Gregory's contorted grimace and a potent smell of stale urine. Pulling on the Posey, a restraint often used to keep agitated patients from harming themselves or others, Mr. Gregory reminded me of a child in a harness anxious to flail his arms and legs freely about. His hospital gown was untied and hoisted above his hips, revealing a freshly changed diaper.

"Hello, Mr. Gregory," I began, trying my best to overcome the bells and whistles blasting from the game show on the TV. "My name is Gretchen and I'm a chaplain here at the hospital."

"Hi," he muttered under his breath, looking every which way except at me.

"Do you mind if I have seat for a minute?" I asked.

"You can sit for *ten* minutes!" he replied, choosing to take my question literally and, in turn, to place himself "one up" on me. As

I pulled up a chair and turned down the TV, I noticed that the room was empty of flowers and cards, yet littered with pieces of tissue and stains from urine, blood, and other excretions. Understaffed, and survivors of the hospital's most recent cost-cutting measures, it appeared that the nurses were unable to provide their usual vigilant care. I suspected that the condition of Mr. Gregory's room suggested more than limited nursing resources, however. In addition, it reflected the patient's compromised condition—both medically and emotionally. With Mr. Gregory, I sensed that the disarray of his room was yet another cry for help from the hidden part of him that no longer seemed to matter to anyone else.

"So you're a . . . chaplain?" he grumbled, looking at me suspiciously.

"Yes, I am. Do you know what a chaplain is?" I asked, regretting my question the very second it came out. I needed to remind myself that even though certain aspects of Mr. Gregory's appearance and behavior reminded me of a child, I was not talking to one. I knew that if I talked down to Mr. Gregory, he would feel diminished in relationship to me—below me. I imagined he had already been pushed into such a pit numerous times.

"Yes, I know what a chaplain is!" he retorted, kicking me back into line.

"Oh, good," I replied, trying to repair the damage. "Some people don't."

We sat in silence for a few minutes, and then I, in my discomfort, chose to dig myself deeper into the hole of my assumptions.

"So you must be frustrated to be in the hospital," I offered, imposing on him what would be my own reaction to his situation.

"No, I'm *not* frustrated!" he replied in a frustrated tone.

"Oh, okay. I'm glad to hear you're not frustrated," I responded, realizing that frustrated or not, his emotions were only valuable to him if he was the one to claim them. He needed to be the one to say how he felt, not me. In fact, no longer able to walk, control his bladder, or do much of anything for himself, expressing his thoughts and emotions was probably one of the few things he could still do independently. And I, just like the multitude of others whose intentions were to help him, was falling into the trap of denying him the very right to help himself.

"So you're a chaplain . . ." he repeated. I wondered what inside of him was causing him to fixate on my title. Did he have a bad experience in the church in the past? Did I not fit his image of a chaplain? Did he assume my visit meant he was going to die? Whatever it was, I decided that I would just go right along with it, allowing him the rare freedom of coming up with his own conclusions.

"Yes, I came by because I wanted to let you know that I care about you," I offered, trying to get past my title to who I really am: someone who cares and devotes her time to expressing it.

"Oh," Mr. Gregory replied with a certain degree of resolution in his voice. He gradually stopped pulling on his Posey, as if he no longer felt the need to fight it.

Suddenly, a plump and jubilant black woman appeared with his lunch, placing it on the tray table in front of him. Part of me was relieved to have an activity to focus on, something to soothe my deceptive need to lead the visit to my own destination. Another part of me was disappointed by the interruption, however, for just as I was starting to provide a safe place for Mr. Gregory to assert his own needs and desires, I was finding yet again that God's hospitable spirit was all the more present. In any case, though, I also knew that God's transforming power could not be blocked by the arrival of a lunch tray.

Mr. Gregory grabbed the top of the bun on his sloppy joe and took a giant bite out of it. As he chewed, a piece of bun protruded from his lips, eventually dropping to the floor. He then tackled the green beans, one flying from his fork to under the bed like a slingshot. The neat and tidy part of me longed to clean up the mess, but I resisted the urge, for deep down I knew that to do so would only serve as another reminder of his helpless state. Besides, the call to be still in the messes of life would be good for me also. I thought of my husband, John, with a smile in my heart. "You gettin' all organized?" he often teases me, as I race to unpack, do laundry, and sort through mail immediately after we return from a trip. Little did Mr. Gregory know that through his lousy eating skills, he was teaching me that life's messes aren't always something to be hastily remedied.

"Will you hand me the peaches?" Mr. Gregory suddenly asked, pointing to the far corner of the tray. I picked up the little yellow dish of fruit and placed it into his shaking hand, along with a clean fork with which to eat them. Mr. Gregory accepted the peaches, but pushed away the fork I offered and then reached for a spoon.

"I guess a spoon works better, huh?" I said, knowing that his utensil selection had far more to do with his longing for respect than his ability to eat peaches.

After Mr. Gregory had finished eating, he pushed his tray away, leaned back into his chair, and let out a sigh. "That was good," he muttered, followed by a blunt burp. I wondered when the last time was that he had dined with another instead of being abandoned or force-fed. Perhaps that day's lunch was the most nourishing meal he had ingested in a long time.

Mr. Gregory and I sat in silence for several minutes, slowly digesting the time we were spending together. He started to nod off, his limp neck yielding to the random jerks of his heavy head. As I looked at him overwhelmed in a peaceful sort of surrender, it was hard to believe that he was the same man whose relentless screeches could be heard throughout the ward just an hour earlier. Somehow, he had entered rest; somehow, he had received what he needed instead of demanding what he didn't need. And I was learning that in allowing Mr. Gregory the freedom to be himself, his defenses disintegrated like wet sandstone, making way for fertile ground in which genuine intimacy could grow. And through the divine direction of this process, I was no longer an enemy, but a friend; no longer a mere visitor, but a guest; and no longer a stranger, but a companion.

Noting that Mr. Gregory would likely be soon sound asleep, I gently touched him on his shoulder to notify him of my departure. He stirred, looking up at me in a foggy gaze. "Well, if you gotta go, you gotta go," he whispered in response, again seeking the control that the rest of his life lacked. I smiled inside, knowing that what appeared to be a cranky retort was really a temporary coping mechanism, for he had already lost too much in his life to relive acute grief over and over again. As is so often the case, Mr. Gregory's response had little to do with me, but instead found its roots in the culmination of experiences stored up within his heart and mind.

"Would you like to have a prayer before I leave?" I asked, knowing full well that the man of frank responses would let me know what he wanted.

"You can," he replied quietly. At first his words confused me, as they implied a certain ambiguity. But then I realized that on a deeper level, Mr. Gregory was giving me permission to approach the part of him he spent so much time protecting, and that his hesitant words were the only way he knew how to do this.

I offered my hand to Mr. Gregory, and he firmly grasped it with both of his hands. He seemed to have jumped at the opportunity for touch, as if it didn't come around very often, except in the form of a needle or baby wipe.

Mr. Gregory and I bowed our heads, and I, as he had, surrendered, allowing the Spirit to come. As is often the case, I experience prayer as a place of active rest, for God's truth and love seem to emanate from my heart in a way that they cannot from my lips alone. Feeling grounded in such a refuge, I closed our prayer with words I felt welling up in my heart. "And thank you, Lord, for Mr. Gregory and for blessing me so richly through him."

As I got up to leave, I noticed Mr. Gregory was staring into his lap in an attempt to hide a cascade of tears. "Thank you," he uttered in a wobbly voice.

"You're welcome," I replied distinctly, trusting that he would come to see that his gift of thanks, a very gift of himself, had been truly received.

23

Living in Love

It is easy to fall into the trap of thinking that my pastoral care ministry ends the moment I leave the hospital. After a day of emotionally draining visits, I find myself relieved to get in my car, turn on the stereo, and let my favorite tunes permeate my mind while I drive home, my thoughts wandering anywhere, everywhere, and nowhere at the same time. My need for such "down time" is understandable, even necessary. However, the temptation is to let my mind continue to roam endlessly into a stale trance of self-absorption, denying myself the privilege of being moved by the Spirit into further creative purpose. I am reminded of the law of thermodynamics: things naturally fall apart when there is no force to keep them bonded in a fluid and ever-changing unity.

Pastoral care is not just my job. It is my vocation, my way of life. It is not a profession whose course I can direct, but rather a divine adventure in which I am willing to partake. I cannot *do* pastoral care where, when, and how *I* want; I can only *be* pastoral care where, when, and how *God* wants. My dependence on the Holy Other to do His work enables me to approach Him with open arms and an expectant heart, through which, and *only* through which, I am filled with His amazing ways of compassion, grace, wisdom, and love. To be a recipient of such blessings is not without its costs, however, costs which come in the form of humbling experiences that serve to call me back to the sacred place of service from which I so often flee.

Such a humbling experience recently befell me. In retrospect, I see that it was no different from any other encounter in that it involved two sacred people in a sacred place at a sacred time, for God is alive in all He has created. However, I was not wearing my lenses of truth at the time, and therefore I initially met the opportunity to take part in divine activity with resistance. Instead of "Yes, Lord, I choose to offer your love," I found myself thinking, "No, Lord, what about me? I need love." Little did I know then that my intense desire for love was to be met in giving it away from the deep well that God had already placed within me.

God's humbling reminder did not come to pass at the hospital, but rather at home. And no, it was not with a patient, but rather with my husband. Yes, my husband. "You mean he needs care, too?" I found myself asking, immediately embarrassed by the fact that the very one who needs my love the most is also the very one to whom I so often fail to show it.

It was 8:30 on a Wednesday night. I took a shower and put on my bathrobe, and then finally resigned myself to transferring the crusty leftovers from the oven to the fridge. A few minutes later, John walked through the door, thirty-six hours after he had initially walked out of it. His lab coat, its pockets characteristically stuffed with countless admission notes, several reference booklets, and a stethoscope, weighed him down like a waterlogged blanket. And his book bag, filled with last month's unopened mail, dirty scrubs, and empty Tupperware, only added to his burden. "It was a long night," he said with a sigh of relief. I took his bag and car keys, oblivious to the fact that he had much more to unload. If only he had the energy . . . if only he had the time . . . if only I would offer him a place for this time.

John took a long-awaited shower while I poured him a tall glass of water and transferred the tired spaghetti onto a plate. He wearily came to the table and ate quickly and hastily, his hunger as ravenous as his desire to climb into bed. I sat down next to him, babbling the events of the last two days quicker than he could digest them: the latest update on the maple floors to be installed in our new house; the challenging visit I had had with a woman whose grief was manifested in violent screams and forceful punches into pillows; the telephone conversation with my sister during which I didn't know how to respond to her words of anger and hurt. I spoke not only about what had happened, but also about the thoughts and emotions the events had stirred up inside of me. John listened, his sleepy eyes about to find their rest in a bed of spaghetti. I waited, my lonely and anxious heart longing for the emotional connection that he could not give. Little did I know then that his silent response was really a call to the Love that already resided within me, a Love whose healing power can only be received when I choose to freely give it away.

I crawled into bed next to John, my heart choosing the unrest of resentment instead of the rest of compassion. I was so overwhelmed by my own need for love that I was looking for it everywhere except inside myself. Unable to sleep, I got up and sought an activity to cover up the pain: cleaning. Instead of attempting to make sense of the mess of emotions crying out to be acknowledged within me, I scrubbed the toilet, did the laundry, unloaded the dishwasher, and mopped the floors. If I could not be loveable, I could at least be useful.

In the wee hours of the morning, I climbed back into bed, physically exhausted from the scrubbing, wiping, and folding. Somehow, my frantic episode of cleaning had brought me to a place in which the emptiness inside was tolerable. My well of nervous energy had run dry, and I had no choice but to be still. Energiless and still—just like the one who slept beside me, breathing in and out with the trust of a baby in a mother's womb. In his peaceful state of surrender, John invited me to go to the exact place from which I had fled: to my heart, to the seat of all my feelings, emotions, and thoughts, to the place that only God can contain.

John, my precious partner of four years, is a third-year resident in Internal Medicine. For the last seven years of his life, he has devoted his time to the accumulation of medical knowledge and its application to those who seek its cures. On a daily basis, he is expected to play God, only to feel inadequate with the rude reminder that he is not. It has been a long and arduous journey for John: from memorizing cranial nerves and metabolic pathways; to flopping into bed at one o'clock in the morning after his first day as an intern, dreading what additional misery was to come in the days and years ahead; to having his beeper stolen by a patient with schizophrenia on a typically stressful day of ceaseless demands.

The journey has also been difficult for me. I, just like his patients, find myself demanding his love, care, and attention: precious commodities that he can't even find time to give to himself, let alone to myself and others. "You know," he said the other night with hints of both relief and sadness, "I haven't even had time to reflect on my own life over the past several years." His simple words of observation unexpectedly ushered my heart from a place of selfish yearning to a place of open compassion. Apparently, I was not as alone as I thought, for just like me, John also harbors feelings of loneliness and emptiness. We are intimately connected in our weariness, in our needs for renewal, in our humanness, in our needs for each other. We are in the same boat, and together we need to row and rest, rest and row, not toward each other, but toward God; not for each other, but for God.

I have learned, and continue to learn, that it is not in making demands on John that my needs for love are met; rather, it is through welcoming his own language of love to speak freely in the home of my heart. In looking beyond my own notions of love, I am freed to see its plethora of expressions in John: in the sharing of his frustrations after a rough day at the hospital; in his closing of the bedroom closet doors at night so the "scary monsters" won't gobble me up; in the daily morning hug and kiss that precede any activity, even putting on his glasses. In receiving John, the John shaped by the hands of the Divine, I offer to him God's love and affirmation. And in offering God's love and affirmation to him, I know God's love for and affirmation of me.

God's call to put my own perceived needs aside and to seek to meet those of John is not always a successful endeavor on my part. Sometimes my desire to return to Eden instead of traveling farther along the road of consciousness sucks me from the carpet of life like a vacuum cleaner. "Being a Christian is too hard!" I yelled the other night, while lying in a puddle of misery on the living room floor. "I hate all the struggles and uncertainties I have! I wish I could just ignore them!" Ironically, it is often during these times of rage that God's grace comes alive to me through John. Sometimes he just listens, allowing me a safe place to act out my temper tantrum of sorts. Other times he tells me that he cares, but that he cannot be there for me at that moment. In his humble self-awareness, he reminds me that he is not God, and offers me the healing perspective that sometimes my struggles need to be mine and mine alone. Yes, to live in love is to be open to its various expressions.

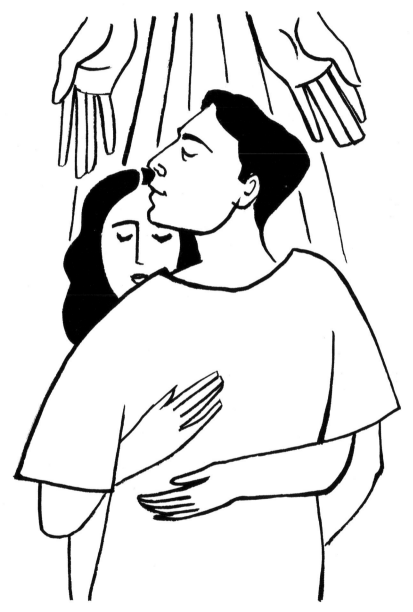

©1999 Michael O'Neill McGrath, OSFS

How awesome it is to be allowed to partake in the divine process of love, not just at home with John, and not just at the hospital with patients, but with anyone God sends my way. I am eternally invited to offer God's grace to all, and in doing so, I am blessed with numerous opportunities to receive it. In the mystery of each individual around me lies a unique glimpse of God's immanent presence, if I am willing to see it. And with each glimpse of God in another, I feel my heart overflow with love, for it is in welcoming God that I can find His true home in my heart.

24

Looking Back Through New Lenses

"I'm really not a very religious man," Mr. Jefferson said, as if such a confession exempted him from any meaningful conversation.

"That's okay. You don't have to be," I replied, appreciative of his frankness. As I sat down next to him, I noticed he was wringing his hands as if they were wet dishrags and clenching his facial muscles as if they were keeping his face from falling to the floor. He looked worried. It appeared as though something was weighing heavily on his mind that he was hesitant to share. I tried to allow myself to be a calm presence, a safe place for him to open up and be himself. I knew I was walking on holy ground.

"This is the fifth time this has happened." He finally broke the silence.

"It sounds like you've been through a lot," I reflected, hoping to provide an opportunity for him to share more about his predicament.

"Yes. And today I'm having surgery," he confided. "I'm waiting to have them pick me up."

"Hmm . . . How are you feeling about having surgery?" I asked, hoping to get beyond the mere facts of the situation.

"Well, it's either that or die," he stated bluntly, looking at me briefly yet intensely, straight into my eyes.

"So you're feeling that there's not much choice involved, huh?" I scrambled for the right words in response to his statement. I wanted to try to be supportive of his confronting the situation honestly.

"Yep, no choice." Mr. Jefferson stared intensely down at his hands, continuing to tug at them as if the frantic activity was the only thing that would keep him from a nervous breakdown. "Maybe he *needs* to have a nervous breakdown," I thought to myself, envisioning myself struggling to tie the anxious man's hands behind his back so that he could vent his feelings in a more productive way. But then I remembered he was about to have surgery—probably not the best timing for an emotional crisis.

"My wife . . . she had a stroke and she's been sick since." Mr. Jefferson slowly began to open up about the numerous concerns I suspected were dominating his mind. "I've been taking care of her," he continued. "But now I can't." I listened intently, reflecting on the significant number of losses this elderly man was facing: his health, his independence, his sense of usefulness, his wife, his relationship with her. His world was falling apart and he couldn't do a thing about it. Neither could I.

I felt a familiar sense of inadequacy rush over me. I wanted to help this man, but I couldn't. I was powerless. Then I remembered what I have learned over and over again, but can never seem to adhere to: that the greatest gift I can give is my presence, my concern, *myself*. Yes, the hardest but most meaningful gifts to give are the ones we cannot touch or buy, for they actually require us to give up a part of ourselves for another. But it is in doing this that we are able to make room for what others have to offer us.

"Everyone in my family—they are all so wonderful." Mr. Jefferson spoke as if they were encapsulated in a distant dream. "My two sons are taking care of the farm, and my daughter is taking care of my wife. I just don't know what I would do without them." Mr. Jefferson appeared to be temporarily consumed by some dramatic insight, as if he had realized for the first time how much he loved his family. Maybe he had.

"I can see that your family means a lot to you," I reflected.

Mr. Jefferson nodded forcefully. Then he suddenly buried his face in his hospital gown and sobbed. He seemed to be feeling a love and appreciation he had never felt before. Now that the possibility of losing his life—in addition to the multitude of other losses he was experiencing—had become real, Mr. Jefferson was coming to recognize how important his family was to him. "And it took a fifth heart attack and a surgery. God is in this darkness," I thought to myself.

Mr. Jefferson and I sat in silence for awhile. He was sitting motionless in the bedside chair, staring off into space. I wondered what thoughts were capturing him in such a state of reverie. My mind came up with several scenarios. Perhaps Mr. Jefferson was reflecting on lost opportunities to tell his wife how much he loved her, back when she was in a state of mind to understand his sentiment. Maybe he was regretting the nights that he worked on the farm until sundown instead of tucking the children in bed. Or perhaps he was looking ahead into the future, wondering if he would be able to provide for his family as he had for so many years. My speculations knew no limits until I suddenly realized how futile they really were. In my heart of hearts, I knew that the details of Mr. Jefferson's past didn't matter as much as the soul searching they were now provoking in him.

I sat in amazement at the sacred moment in which I was blessed to partake: me, merely a stranger, just a lay chaplain who looks like a teenager playing grown up, a wayward follower of Jesus, a young woman trying to find God in all those she meets; and Mr. Jefferson, an honest man ripe with genuine emotion, a seasoned traveler finding greater purpose in the twists and turns of his lifelong journey, a fellow sinner on the pilgrimage to the throne of grace, a solitary individual finding his true home in the hearts of others. I believed Mr. Jefferson was closer to God than he thought. I guess humility works that way.

Somehow an offer for prayer seemed appropriate. "Would you like to have a prayer, Mr. Jefferson, or would you prefer not to?" I was careful, perhaps too careful, not to push this man who acknowledged no special connection with God.

"Yes, that would be good," he accepted. "I want to pray that I'll get better again so I can take care of my wife."

"How about getting better for yourself?" I wanted to ask. But somehow, the question didn't feel right. I sensed that Mr. Jefferson was beyond himself, a place to which he had inadvertently avoided venturing all his life. Little did he know that this is the direction his heart had longed to go all along.

25

Always in Process

"Don't you play smart with me, Justin!" the nurse hollered as she walked out of the thirteen-year-old's room. I knew from that moment on that the visit would be a challenging one. "Oh, no, what am I getting myself into?" I thought to myself as I knocked on the boy's door, wishing I could round only on those rare patients whose delightful demeanors deceive me into believing that they are the only ones worthy of care.

"Hi, Justin. My name is Gretchen and I'm a chaplain. I'm here to see how you're feeling today." My typical introduction, perhaps overly intrusive in retrospect, felt like the kickoff to a football game. I punted as best as I knew how, and then waited to see where my ball would land.

"I'm okay," Justin responded in a barely audible voice. He sat in the bedside chair, slouching to such a degree that his tired eyes were just peering over the half-eaten breakfast tray in front of him. With his head resting sideways on the armrest, he looked painfully adolescent: disinterested, lonely, insecure, and bored. Complications from his sickle-cell anemia had landed him in the hospital for eight days.

"Do you mind if I sit down for a moment?" I asked, anticipating another apathetic response.

"You can," he said with a sigh and a blank stare. "But just don't ask me lots of questions." His response caught me off guard as I immediately recognized that this sly teenager was able to see through my formal introduction with the ease of a chess master. Apparently, I was just another "staff person," and he, a veteran patient who knew the hospital routine all too well for his tender age.

"Sounds like a deal," I replied, knowing that the pledge would be a difficult one for my restless spirit to keep. We sat together in silence for several minutes, Justin staring out the window with the purpose of a roaming cow, and me sporadically perusing the room with the fluidity of a buzzing bumblebee. If it weren't for his limp arm and multiple IV lines protruding from it, I could have been mistaken for the patient.

"You can ask me questions," he finally blurted. "I can tell you want to." His comment served to heighten my anxiety and erect my defenses.

"Not really," I lied. "Is there anything that you would like to talk about?" As my words floated through the air, I realized the absurdity of my actions. I had denied my desire to ask questions, only to then ask one. "This kid has me all figured out," I thought to myself, feeling like a diary torn open for all of the world to read. In retrospect, I see that during that time, I felt what it was to be a patient: exposed, vulnerable, and uncertain. Perhaps Justin was projecting a glimpse of his own life onto mine. Unfortunately, I was too absorbed in my own feelings to be available to his.

Justin adeptly ignored my question, giving me the grace for a second chance, yet at the same time, winding my will around his finger with the facility of a seasoned seamstress. "Will you straighten up those things over there?" he suddenly asked, pointing to the array of items on his windowsill. Straighten—a word that signifies what he lacked in his own life and sought to obtain in the world around him: structure, order, and control.

"Sure," I replied, relieved that I could finally do something in the midst of not knowing what to do with myself. In response to his commands, I turned the clock radio toward his chair, placed the stuffed bear in the gift bag so that its head was peeping out, and lined the get-well cards in an orderly row. Made to feel useful, I was actually disappointed to finish the task. To my relief, however, he watered my false need to be busy as if it were a sun-scorched flower.

"Will you clear my tray?" he asked with the expectation of a king to his servant. I immediately agreed, quickly and efficiently transferring his tray to the cafeteria cart in the hallway.

"Will you get my Walkman out of the closet?" he then demanded in the deceptive form of a question. Just as I was about to agree to the chore, it occurred to me with the sudden clarity of a

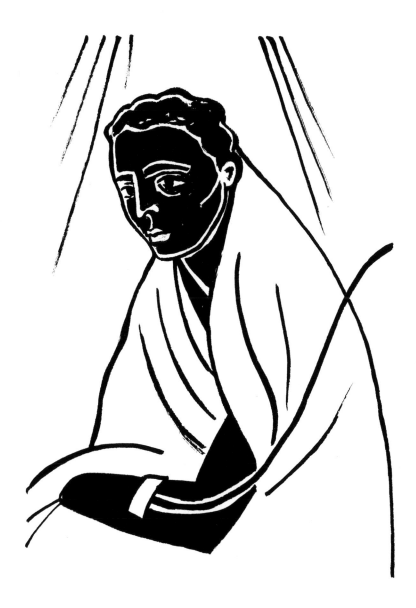

struck match that I had become the maid instead of the chaplain. Yes, this boy of half my age was a master of manipulation. He had me right where he wanted me, and I was ashamed to admit it.

Confined to the grasp of my human nature, I then attempted to turn the tides of our power struggle of sorts. "I think you can get your Walkman yourself," I said in the friendliest tone I could muster. Meanwhile, I took pleasure in my thoughts of revenge, imagining myself saying "Get it yourself, buddy!" or stuffing the Walkman down his throat. Yes, I was a chaplain, a chaplain clothed in the mess of her own humanity.

Justin then pursued another avenue of manipulation, masked in the guise of self-pity. "That nurse won't let me get back into bed. I hate this chair. It makes me hurt more."

"That sounds frustrating," I offered, sensing a glimmer of hope that our visit could be taking a step toward productivity.

"Will you tell her that you think I need to get back in bed?"

With Justin's final ploy for control and attention, I snapped. "You know, Justin, sometimes you gotta do what you don't wanna do," I retorted. My threshold of tolerance for his uncooperative behavior had been reached. Little did I know then that my threshold had been so low that it had never even existed. In fact, I didn't give Justin a chance from the moment I walked in the door.

Looking back on my visit with Justin, I am embarrassed, disappointed, and discouraged: embarrassed that I call myself a chaplain when I am not always faithful to the role; disappointed that I am capable of harming others in the name of help; and discouraged that I so often unintentionally let my own "stuff" get in the way of being truly available to others. Instead of responding to the feelings behind Justin's behavior, I reacted to the behavior itself. I was caught up in my own false need for control: in my subconscious subscription to the view that children are to obey and be subject to discipline at all times, a way of life that fed my own craving for stability and predictability when I was young. When Justin didn't match up with my expectations for a "good child," I felt it was my duty to "set him straight." Our time together then transformed itself into a power struggle, a duel between a child and a childish adult. If only I had been able to recognize that what needed my attention was not his behavior but rather the array of feelings that were hiding behind it.

As I reflect on the time I spent with Justin, I recognize that his manipulative manners may have been his survival mechanism, his way of coping with a debilitating disease that was robbing him of the carefree childhood that others take for granted. Sickle-cell anemia is a painful and progressive illness that knows no cure, leaving its sufferers subject to permanent tissue damage caused by frequent blockages of blood supply to different parts of the body. Now that a recent stroke had left his right arm helpless, he had only to wait for what would befall him next: another intense wave of abdominal pains that the medication didn't seem to help, a limp leg that he could no longer walk on. The various possibilities were endless, but they all shared one thing in common: a life sentence of uncertainty that served to remind Justin of his powerless state like a slap in the face.

Ironically, we all share in Justin's condition, only our transitory illusions of independence and self-sufficiency lead us to believe otherwise. Looking back, I see that Justin and I had a lot more in common than I was willing to admit. Both tired of being pulled with the unpredictable tides of life, we sought the control over each other that we couldn't achieve for ourselves. Justin and I were hurting in the same place. If only I had been open to this truth at the very time it cried out to be heard, then perhaps Justin and I could have been allies instead of enemies. If only I had asked Justin what he didn't like about questions instead of running from the subject matter in an attempt to protect my own pride; if only I had offered a safe place for him to share his feelings about being disabled instead of playing servant; if only I could have been available to his feelings instead of ignoring them alltogether; if only I could have accepted his frustration with being in the hospital instead of telling him that he needed to do what the nurse told him. If only . . .

"Oh, to do it over again!" These words have flooded my mind after countless pastoral care visits. Each and every time, I am reminded of how difficult it is to minister to another without letting my own issues get in the way. The culmination of my life's experiences and all of the thoughts and emotions they have brought forth modify my views of the world around me like an ever-changing lens. Sometimes I can see more clearly, enabling me to come to know God's immanent presence in new and amazing ways. Other times, all I see is a blur, detracting from the beautiful vision that God would have for me. But I take great comfort in the fact that however I relate to the world around me—whether with the clarity of divine insight or with the blinders of my human nature—God goes with me. The pleasure that I sense from God when I have shown His wise and authentic love to others continually sets my soul on fire, moving me ever-forward in sacred service. And His grace surrounds me like a warm blanket when I have cast my own crooked shadow upon His light, leading me farther along the eternal path of healing restoration.

—26—

At a Distance

Mr. Reynolds had called for a chaplain on that rainy February morning, and to this day, I'm still not sure why. The sixty-two-year-old Episcopalian was recovering from a pulmonary embolism, a blood clot to his lung that could have killed the otherwise healthy man if left untreated. Despite the trauma of the last few days, however, Mr. Reynolds projected the image of a smooth-talking, self-assured salesman. "I'm just great!" he immediately proclaimed when I asked him how he was feeling that day.

"You're an Episcopalian, too, right?" the burly man asked me as I stood at the foot of the bed looking for a place to sit down. Internally, I winced at the familiar question about my religion, as I find that preoccupation with denominational similarities and differences tend to deter from the fact that we are all children of God.

"Yes, as a matter a fact, I am," I replied. Despite my preference for looking beyond the divisions we make among ourselves, I hoped the commonality would foster a connection between the two of us.

"Great!" he shouted with a laugh and a swoosh of the fist. "So is my trooper of a son, Mark," he continued, pointing to the frail man sitting in the opposite corner of the room. I had not even noticed Mark before his father brought attention to him, in a manner that suggested he were still in the Boy Scouts. As the visit progressed, I sensed that their relationship had always worked this way, and therefore was not surprised that the younger man had chosen to remain at a distance. I wondered, if given the chance, how Mark would elect to present himself.

"Yep, I've been an Episcopalian all my life," Mr. Reynolds began a lengthy tirade, ignoring his son's response to his introduction. "Not really," Mark had mumbled under his breath, rejecting the label of an Episcopalian. Even though the thirty-something computer analyst spoke with the purpose of an oozing slug, I sensed that his few words were reverberating with deafening force inside his head. Part of me identified with Mark, as I, too, have longed to tell others who I am instead of living according to the images that they would have for me.

"They should have never changed to the 1979 prayer book, you know," Mr. Reynolds continued, shaking his head in disapproval. "The 1928 was much better. All of my friends in the diocese agree with me. What do you think?"

Before I had the chance to respond to the question, which seemed to emerge from the confines of his restless spirit, Mr. Reynolds continued his harangue. "Well, let me tell you what Professor So-and-so down at VTS (a local seminary) thinks . . ." Then with the urgency of an overflowing toilet, the man with diarrhea of the mouth slightly diverted the course of his monologue. "For goodness sake, you look young. You must be a student down at VTS. Is that right! Do you know . . . ?"

Standing at the foot of his bed like a lone flamingo, I listened to Mr. Reynolds, and it occurred to me that he was not interested in what anyone else had to say except himself. He was looking to dictate his philosophy, not share his fears; to proclaim his doctrine, not discuss his doubts; to assert his tenets, not learn from his trials; to impress the chaplain, not inquire of God's presence with her. Having faced the reality of death and the fragility of life, I sensed that Mr. Reynolds now felt the need to construct a fortress of control that deep down he knew he didn't have. To pretend he had power was the closest he could get to actually possessing it. Therefore, he would hear only what he wanted to hear and see only what he wanted to see. This scenario is a familiar one—one we all visit from time to time when difficult circumstances threaten our illusions of self-sufficiency.

After about fifteen minutes of nonstop talk, Mr. Reynolds seemed to run out of things to say, perhaps subconsciously realizing that his ploy for control had been discovered. He suddenly looked up at me expectantly, as if to say "What now, Chaplain?"

"What can I do to help you, Mr. Reynolds?" I finally asked after a minute of silence.

He looked at me in an air of confusion and uncertainty, perhaps allowing himself to visit these foreign feelings for the first time in a long while. He cleared his throat several times, struggling to maintain the mask of self-assurance that he had worked so hard to project. "Aren't you supposed to know that?" he finally asked in desperation.

"Well, we could talk, we could pray, we could sit together, or I could leave." I presented the options clearly and succinctly, and then awaited his reply.

"How about pray!" he suggested with the certainty of a coin toss. I gladly accepted his proposal, albeit with a certain degree of suspicion as to his motives. Hoping to promote more intimacy among the three of us, I invited Mark to join. He agreed in a sort of resignation and moved his chair toward the bedside, as if he had nothing better to do. Unable to locate another chair, I decided to sit on the edge of the bed, something I have been taught not to do for fear of sitting on a needle or invading a patient's space. Weary of the rigid boundaries that were dominating our interactions, however, I was anxious to move on from the superficiality. Looking back, however, I see that the need for connection was more mine than Mr. Reynolds' or Mark's. Yes, the two men had oodles of issues crying out to be acknowledged, hiding behind coping mechanisms that while effective, could only be temporary. I suspected, however, that they would be free to remove their masks when, and only when, they were free to leave them on.

"What would you like to be sure to include in prayer?" I asked, making a final offer for anything real. The two men just looked at each other and shrugged their shoulders, apparently not ready to scratch the surface of their hearts' desires. Part of me longed to force this information, to skillfully extract it like a dentist removing a wisdom tooth. But then I realized that to do so would only be to distort its progress, like inducing a pregnant woman whose child is not ready to be born.

"How about I just pray?" I finally proposed. Mr. Reynolds and his son looked at me with a sigh of relief. Watching their identical responses, I wondered if they realized how similar they were in spite of their differences. While they kept themselves at a distance from each other, they were really walking hand in hand along the same rocky road of living in relationship.

I offered my hands to Mr. Reynolds and Mark, suggesting we form a prayer circle. The two men hesitated, but then quickly accepted, even if only to get the moment over with. To hold hands is a powerful statement of unity, interdependence, and trust. I suspected that Mark and his father had rarely visited these foreign feelings together in the past. Then again, perhaps they had in some way that I could not understand, in some way that was comprehensible only in the context of the unique father and son relationship they shared. I am frequently humbled by the continual realization that intimacy is not limited to overt expressions of emotion as I so often experience it to be.

"Dear Lord . . ." I began to pray. My exact words elude me as I write, although I remember that they were characterized by a reserved formality. I had my own specific ideas of how each man needed to be prayed for, but I sensed that to simply throw my spiritual prescription at them like an unsolicited flyer would probably do more harm than help. I took comfort in the fact that God was touching the parts of themselves that they could not. Like a faithful shepherd, God gently pursues us no matter how far we stray.

As I closed my prayer, the two men quickly released hands as if the act had been a painful one. In a sense it probably had, as the open gesture had most likely served to knock on doors that had long been sealed shut. To answer the call for communion would be to surrender the separateness that fed the insatiable human hunger to be one's own God.

"Thanks for coming," Mr. Reynolds suddenly blurted, his typically voluminous words reducing themselves to just a few. "You have a good day now." Apparently, the roller coaster of a visit had overwhelmed him, especially the last few twists and turns that had come upon him unexpectedly. It was time for Mr. Reynolds to withdraw into his cave of control, a place of protection that would serve its purpose if and when he would find the courage to venture from it on a regular basis.

As I looked in the man's eyes to bid him farewell, I noticed a few teardrops rolling down his cheeks. Part of me wanted to hug him, to reach out to him, to ask him what was wrong. But deep down I knew that nothing was wrong, that he was exactly where he needed to be: at a distance. Not a distance that erected permanent walls, but a distance that allowed temporary boundaries as necessary. Mark simply gazed at his father in a dreamlike state. Perhaps he was coming to know a part of his father he had never met before. And perhaps he was beginning to recognize a part of himself in this man he had always tried so hard to be different from.

Another Side of Me

Mr. Turner presented me with one of the most difficult challenges I have ever faced in pastoral care. Not because of any horrific situation in which I found him, and not because of any combative demeanor he exhibited, but rather because of the cascade of uncomfortable feelings our visits together unleashed in me. Uncomfortable feelings: feelings of vulnerability and weakness, feelings of exposure, feelings of shame, feelings I wanted to run away from and pretend were not there. Even as I write, I feel a pit in my stomach, reminding me of how threatened I felt, and even continue to feel, by this man who seemed to shine a flashlight directly into a part of myself I had never before known was there.

I first met Mr. Turner on one of the medical wards. After being admitted to the hospital for multiple head wounds and a broken arm, the forty-six-year-old Christian had requested that a chaplain come for prayer. He was accompanied in his room by a young woman whose eyes were glued to a muted Jerry Springer on the television. "The sitter is for Mr. Turner's safety," the nurses had said. Apparently, he had been found wandering the city streets with a bloody head, and it was unclear as to whether his injuries were the result of an attack or self-inflicted.

Our initial visit was brief. This was to my relief, as Mr. Turner's bruised and lacerated face and the smell of raw flesh and sweat that emanated from it made me nauseous. Trying to conceal my urge to gag, I asked what he would like to include in prayer. "Let's pray that the Lord will give me strength to get through this," he uttered in a feeble voice. As we bowed our heads, I offered my hand, trying my best to ignore the dried blood under his fingernails.

Our time together ended uneventfully. "A pretty routine visit," I remember thinking to myself as I headed back down the hallway.

Since then, I have learned that no visit is simply "routine," at least when God is doing the work.

A few days later, Mr. Turner requested another visit. "He wants to see that 'little chaplain with the long hair,' " the nurse relayed the message. I made my way up to the ward, finding him sitting up in bed no longer accompanied by the sitter, wearing the best smile his crooked mouth would allow. His broken arm was held firmly in a sling, and his swollen face was patched up with gauze bandages. "I'm so glad you came," he immediately opened up upon my arrival, looking up at me longingly. "It meant so much to me when we prayed together the other day. I thought I was going to die." Before I could respond, he immersed me into a sea of compliments. "I think what you do is so wonderful . . ." he commented, his eyes gazing softly into mine. "I sense that you really have an availability to the Holy Spirit," he continued. Before I knew it, I had become the patient, dosing myself with his kind words as if they were life-saving drugs. How comforting it was to be valued, approved of, and accepted.

"Please come back," Mr. Turner proposed after we closed our visit in prayer. I agreed without hesitation, figuring that this kind man with the gentle yet unsophisticated disposition of Yogi Bear would benefit from the additional support. Looking back, I see that my desire to return was not just for him, but also for me.

The next time I saw Mr. Turner, he was on the psychiatric ward. He had mentioned nothing previously of his struggle with bipolar illness, and I, figuring he would share what he wanted to, had not queried the details of his mental health. It did not take me long to realize, however, that his illness dictated the course of his life like a hurricane.

"I have so much to tell you today," he pronounced as I entered his room. I was immediately taken aback by the small space that felt more like a dungeon for solitary confinement than a refuge for peaceful convalescence. The flimsy bare mattress was strewn with dirty linens, bunches of tissue and open books, and the dreary potato sack curtains that attempted to decorate the puny, so called windows were drawn shut. I wondered if the state of his room was any indication of what he felt on the inside: disheveled, confused, dark, and alone.

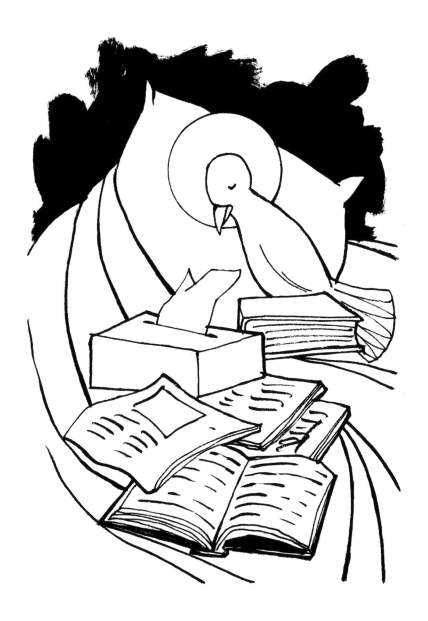

As we both sat down, Mr. Turner immediately launched into a lengthy discourse about his life experiences: his past career in politics, his aspiration to go to seminary, his despair over a recent divorce, his scattered family, and those "close" friends he hadn't talked with in years. He shared with the ease of a mountain stream in the springtime, and I felt honored to be entrusted with the rushing waters of his life. "After I go to seminary, I'm going to run for U.S. Senate," Mr. Turner suddenly proclaimed. "God has told me that this is His plan." I received his somewhat grandiose notion with an appropriate degree of doubt, but deep down, I knew that to challenge his proposal was not what his heart needed. Mr. Turner's perception of reality was different from mine, but it was *his*, and at that moment, that's what seemed to matter the most.

I wondered how many others had shot down Mr. Turner's plans like enemy aircraft, how many had shaken their heads at him in helpless frustration. Too many, I suspected. I sensed that he needed someone he could trust to hear his unusual ideas, someone who was willing to make a detour to join him for a once-in-a-lifetime pilgrimage. It then occurred to me that what he needed was what he had so aptly bestowed upon me during our previous visit: a time and place to be valued, approved of, and accepted.

Mr. Turner continued to unload his thoughts and feelings, one after the other, as if they might disintegrate if he didn't get them out before his impending discharge. The stories, the plans, the memories, the visions, spewed forth like bubbles from a simmering pot of stew. I just sat nodding, smiling, "mm hmming," tasting his strange yet amicable world spoonful by spoonful. On occasion he would ask me a question about my life, and I would respond freely, adding my own sort of savory seasoning to our feast of thoughts and emotions. It was as if Mr. Turner and I had known each other our entire lives, and our conversation was a sort of homecoming.

After an hour or so had passed, Mr. Turner's and my words slowly came to a halt. I felt full but not stuffed, as if I'd just eaten a hearty bowl of morning oatmeal with brown sugar on top. We sat in silence, both profoundly aware that our time together had possessed a rare and blessed resonance. "I wouldn't tell all this to anyone I didn't think of as . . . as a sort of partner," he finally blurted with an awkward laugh. Not to my surprise, I was thinking the same thing, only pretending that I really wasn't. The acknowledgment was an uncomfortable one for me, for never before had I experienced such a connection with another man, except for my husband. Oddly enough, this gift of genuine intimacy was not one I was sure I wanted more than once. Yet there it sat, right before us in that delicate moment, begging to be claimed for what it was, whether with deep yearning or paralyzing dread.

As Mr. Turner and I sat in the awkward aftermath of his straightforward statement, part of me wanted to reach out to hold and be held by him, part of me wanted to run out of the room, and part of me wanted to do both. I opted for the latter, hoping that there could exist a happy medium amid all of my contradictory emotions. We folded our arms around each other in a gentle hug that felt genuine and not contrived, needed and not simply a matter of routine.

"Can I give you a kiss on the cheek?" he asked as we parted. His question took me by surprise and added to the array of emotions already storming my heart and mind. "Sure," I replied quickly, as anxious to get the act out of the way as to enjoy the touch of his lips on my face. He planted a soft peck on my right cheek, and before I knew it I was headed into the hallway, waving good-bye. The "now what?" moment had passed, and I still wasn't sure what exactly I had done with it.

For several days after my last visit with Mr. Turner, I checked the hospital census to see whether he had been discharged as scheduled. Although he had indeed left, he was still in my heart, a reality that I both savored and detested. When I was with Mr. Turner, I felt safe, warm, and at home, yet also vulnerable, out of control, and in unfamiliar territory. "How could I experience all these feelings at the same time?" I remember thinking to myself amid a tirade of other anxious questions. "How could I feel this close to a stranger? Am I being unfaithful to my husband? Should I be thankful for this experience or should I be rebuking it?"

Such questions remain in my head to this day, further explored yet still unanswered. I notice again and again in numerous relationships that whenever I get close to the authentic companionship my heart longs for, I abandon it for fear that I will ruin it, distort it, or lose myself in it. Repeatedly, I pursue intimacy only to pull back on its reins when it touches me where I most need it. Strangely, the line between my spirituality and sexuality is a thin one that keeps me constantly struggling for a balance, for both involve a God-given desire to be whole: to become one, to freely give and freely receive, to fulfill and be fulfilled, to serve and be served, to accept and be accepted, to seek and be sought. The tension between the two serves as a constant reminder of my desire for God, my dependence on Him, and my need for His guidance and grace. "I don't want to have this struggle!" I recently sobbed into my husband's arms, amid what felt like a shameful confession. He just listened and held me, seeming to know that I needed a safe place where even this rattled and uncertain side of me was welcome.

—28—

To Be in Relationship Again

Ms. Adams' illegible scrawl littered the front page of my legal pad, making it look like a tornado had landed on it. I knew that she had intended to put the letters in their correct places, but for me they just spelled out gibberish. Even though I couldn't read her writing, it was clear to me what she was trying to say: I want to communicate, I want to talk, I want to be in relationship again.

The seventy-something woman whom I had come across during my rounds sat limp in her chair like a rag doll, her deep brown eyes staring blankly into the hall at nothing in particular. A recent stroke had rendered her speech and writing skills useless. I could only imagine what was going through her mind. What would it be like, I wondered, to be surrounded by a world that you could no longer reach? The feeling of being attacked and tickled to death as a child by my two older sisters came to mind. Pinned to the floor, I was unable to escape what seemed an endless torture. Maybe this is what Ms. Adams felt like. Probably worse.

Ms. Adams' disabilities didn't keep her from trying to communicate, however. I recall at the beginning of our visit how she slowly and carefully formed sounds with her mouth, sounds which she had intended to be words. "I . . . I . . . I . . . ow . . . ow . . . I ow," she uttered, pursing her lips purposefully and grasping the armrest as if it were the actual source of her labored speech. Every few seconds she would cough and gasp from the nasogastric tube that constantly scratched against her throat. She was funneling all of her energy into this futile attempt to speak. To speak: a skill that I take for granted daily, a skill that she probably once took for granted, too.

Her words made no sense to me; it was as if she was speaking another language. Occasionally, I was able to discern a word or two, but otherwise I was left feeling completely clueless. I so much wanted to be able to understand her, to connect with her in a way that would allow her to participate in life and not just observe it. I felt helpless. We both felt helpless. This is probably one of the few things we shared in common.

After several unsuccessful attempts at communication, I couldn't tell whether my presence was of solace or frustration to her. Was she comforted because I, a mere stranger with no apparent agenda, would choose to spend time with her, an invalid who probably felt as if she had little left to offer? Or was she frustrated that I, someone who had no idea what she was thinking and feeling, was bringing attention to her disabilities that needed no further magnification, as they only served to remind her of her helpless state? The answers to my questions seemed to elude me like burned-out lightbulbs occupying an out-of-reach chandelier. I resorted to what seemed the most reliable method of communication: yes or no questions.

"Ms. Adams," I offered somewhat hesitantly. "I'm going to ask you some yes and no questions. Nod for yes, and shake your head for no," I explained, making my own corresponding gestures.

"Do you want me to leave and let you rest? I want to do what's best for you." She shook her head forcefully.

"Do you want me to stay with you for awhile?" She nodded her head. I was relieved to know what she wanted, but at the same time, somewhat surprised by her response. "Why does she want me to stay?" I pondered. "I can't seem to do anything for her." Then I realized that Ms. Adams didn't want me *to do* anything for her. She didn't want *something*; she wanted *someone*. She wanted me.

Ms. Adams and I continued to sit together, oscillating between stilted efforts at communication and awkward periods of silence. Grappling for a topic of conversation, any topic, I told her about how I hated that nasogastric tube when I was in the hospital, how it tickled my throat like a fly that couldn't be swatted. She nodded ardently, and a tender grin came across her face. It was as if the memory I shared, which felt arbitrary and desperate at the time, had actually served to comfort her somehow. Maybe for the first time since her stroke she didn't feel completely alone.

"You know, Ms. Adams," I offered after another stifling period of silence, a phenomenon whose healing presence continues to gnaw at me like a scab I want to pick. "You have really pretty eyes. They're such a deep brown." My compliment was sincere, yet felt random and contrived, perhaps derived from my own fears of what it would feel like to be in her situation. She seemed to be touched by my words, however, tilting her head to the side as her mouth embraced a vivid smile. I was hoping that my comment would make her feel that she still had something to offer. Yes, she had lost a lot, but not everything. In some ways, I wondered if her tragic situation would actually serve to enable her to find the treasures inside her that the tasks of her more productive days had masked.

The time passed slowly yet purposefully, and I sensed after forty-five paradoxically rich minutes of doing close to nothing, that it was time to close our visit. I asked her if she would like to have a prayer, and she agreed. We bowed our heads and I lifted Ms. Adams to God, giving thanks for her and asking for His peace in her life. After closing our prayer, Ms. Adams nodded her head vigorously, saying "thank you" repeatedly in her own special way: "Ank oo, ank oo." Her words spoke louder and clearer than those of someone with perfect pronunciation.

As we parted, something inside of me longed to stay with Ms. Adams, to try to alleviate her pain, to "fix" her situation, to rescue her from the loneliness that dominated her world . . . something inside of me longed to play God himself. But deep down I knew that I needed to entrust her in all of her brokenness to the One who had made her, to the One who knew the desires of her heart, to the One who felt all that she felt. Yes, God was the only One who could fill her emptiness. And I found joy in realizing that God had used me, with all of my weaknesses and insecurities, to play a small but significant part in that holy process.

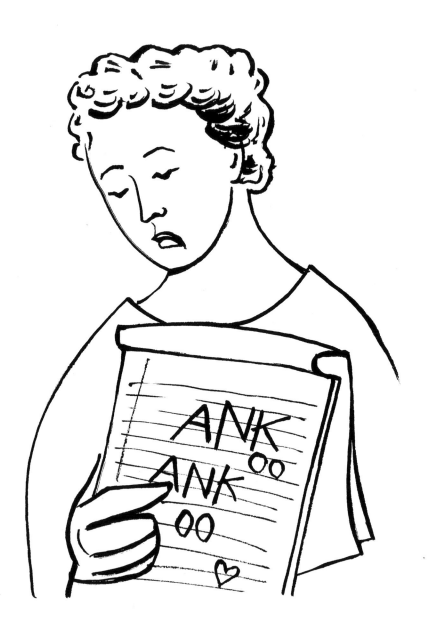

Necessary Friction

It wasn't long after I entered Mr. Brown's room that I wished I hadn't. The 300-pound man with the booming voice intimidated me from the moment I laid eyes on him. And his cranky restless behavior didn't do much to remedy the situation. As I introduced myself, he just stared blankly at the television, flipping the channels with the remote more quickly than he could register what each one was broadcasting. It looked as though he was preoccupied with everything and nothing at the same time. His thick and swollen leg, resembling a gigantic sausage, was held hostage in a large metal contraption.

"Oh, I think someone from your department already came by," he immediately responded after I had introduced myself. "He gave me communion." Mr. Brown's words traveled through the air with the force of a windstorm, making me feel that I could easily be blown right out of the room. Dreading the time I might spend with him, I had no other choice but to plant my feet in the firm foundation of the Lord who I knew had led me there.

"So what are you here to tell me, Chaplain?" he roared.

"Not a good sign," I thought to myself. His question suggested to me from the moment it was posed that we were not off to an optimal start. If this man thought I was here to play drill sergeant, then I obviously had not made the right first impression. Either that, or his past experience with the church was likely to have been more like being in a prison cell than a nurturing retreat. Despite my disadvantageous position, I tried my best to work toward a connection with this man. For this to happen, I sensed that Mr. Brown needed to know that I was here to talk *with* him, not *at* him; to *join* him on his journey, not to *take* him on one.

"I'm not here to tell you anything, really." I stumbled over my words, hoping that they conveyed the message I tried to send. "I'm here for you." Mr. Brown just stared at me looking confused. We sat in silence, not knowing quite what to do with ourselves. Part of me wanted to leave, to abandon the path that appeared destined to go nowhere. But part of me wanted to stay, trusting that God was present in even the most awkward situations.

"What should we talk about?" Mr. Brown threw the question up in the air out of mere desperation.

"Well, I'm here for you, so let's talk about what you would like to talk about." My response was as much based in meeting Mr. Brown's needs as it was in my desire to escape any sense of responsibility for whatever conversation was to come. I hate to be put on the spot, as it forces me to go beyond myself to the place of trust; it forces me to go to God. Yes, I have become adept at running from my very Source, only to realize that He patiently accompanies me wherever I go, simply waiting for me to call upon His name.

"Okay, I have a question for you, Chaplain," Mr. Brown finally blurted with a sense of relief. I just nodded, sensing that he didn't want to talk with me, but just to get answers from me. We both seemed to be pushing each other in just the places we didn't want to go. Yes, God was at work.

"So how do you explain the Trinity, Chaplain?" The question dropped like a bomb, and an "Oh, shit" rolled through my thoughts. I felt as if I was taking a final exam for which I had not studied. The Trinity—one of the most mysterious theological truths, and he wanted *me* to explain it. I wanted to run away from the question, as the concept was not totally clear in my own mind, only I was too ashamed to admit it. I was the chaplain. I was supposed to know this, right? At the same time, I knew that even if I did have the perfect answer, in which case I would be God, it was not my role to spoon feed it to Mr. Brown. Instead, I felt called to lift up his question, trusting that if his searching were genuine, it would come to fruition in its own flawless timing.

"Well, the Trinity is a mysterious concept, God being three in one: the Father, the Son, and the Holy Spirit," I began, resorting to the common denominator of all explanations. "But it doesn't much matter what I think about the Trinity. What matters most is what you think." My response hung in the air for what seemed an eternity. I was not certain of what motives lay behind my brief reply: my own pride or a desire to facilitate Mr. Brown's own seeking. Probably both. In either case, the question prompted us both to examine the very parts of ourselves that we so skillfully ignored. Mr. Brown was forced to look beyond the answers of others to find out how their explanations settled in his own heart and mind. I, on the other hand, was forced to come face to face with my own theology and how to communicate it. Just what did I believe? And how could I offer it to others in a way that made sense?

"Hey, you're taking the easy way out," Mr. Brown replied in response to my challenge. "You're the chaplain. You're supposed to have the complete answer." His line of reasoning poked me right where I didn't want to be touched. It appeared that we both had a way of getting under each other's skin.

"So chaplains are supposed to have all the answers, huh?" I reflected, hoping to shed light on the fact that there was a more reliable Source. At the same time, I felt inadequate and unprepared, like a draft dodger unwilling to venture outside his own country and daily routines. "Always be prepared to give an answer to everyone who asks you to give the reason for the hope that you have. But do this with gentleness and respect." This scripture popped clearly into my mind as if it had been stamped on my forehead.

"Well, you at least have to have an opinion, Chaplain," he continued, prodding me like a cow that wouldn't enter the barn. "Chaplain"—his repetitive use of the title began to annoy me, as I was beginning to feel as if I didn't have command of the vast body of knowledge that it suggested.

"It seems to be awfully important to you to know my opinion," I replied.

"Oh, look at you! You just keep dodging my questions. You're just too much!" He threw his hands up in the air and forced a few chuckles, joking and serious at the same time. I joined in the hesitant spurt of laughter, searching for some rescue from the awkward situation.

The social worker then entered, providing another convenient escape from our banter. "Hi, Mr. Brown," she exclaimed while charging into the room, the pitch of her voice matching the loudness of Mr. Brown's in its intensity. "I need to talk to you about your rehab arrangements. Is this a bad time?" She looked at us both expectantly, pretending to be polite with her question that sought only the accommodation she wanted to hear. I looked to Mr. Brown for his preference, resorting to my usual habit of letting the patient make the decisions.

"Yes, it is. Come back later," he replied bluntly. The social worker raised her eyebrows with shock, and then scurried out of the room like a frightened mouse. I, too, was surprised with Mr. Brown's response, expecting him to jump at the opportunity to kick me out of the room. Strangely, however, we were growing on each other. We both seemed to push each other's buttons, buttons that we didn't want pushed but deep down knew we needed to have pushed. Like two dancing porcupines, we poked one another with our quills, each jab revealing the other's vulnerable bare skin.

After the social worker left, Mr. Brown went into a tirade about her. "She doesn't know what she's doing. She just pretends to be nice. The nurses and doctors are the same way." He shook his head in disgust. I wondered if he was experiencing the same thing in me. Apparently, I wasn't the only one who wasn't good enough for Mr. Brown. In fact, I doubted that *any person* could live up to his standards for competence. No one could give him all of the answers that he wanted; no one could dictate what he needed to discover on his own.

The interruption left us both at a loss for words, and the stifling silence proved to be too much for Mr. Brown to endure. "Well, thanks for coming by," he finally blurted, inviting me to bid him farewell. The sudden request made me feel somewhat confused, disoriented, and left hanging, as if I were riding in a reckless automobile that had come to a screeching halt. Perhaps this was for the better, however, as Mr. Brown and I had already traveled some rough terrain together, and I sensed that we each had our own paths to pursue in the days ahead.

—30—

Empty Before God

"I just . . . I just can't believe that . . . that this is happening to me," Ms. Willis uttered in a shaky voice. Her words came hesitantly, but then settled into the air with great relief, as if she had just pulled one of her own teeth. The thirty-six-year-old African-American woman sat in a restless heap on her bed, staring down at her fiddling fingers.

"You know," she continued, suddenly throwing her arms up into the air, "you hear about this happening to other people, but not to you! You never think it can happen to you!" Her voice took on more force with each word, revealing her anger that seeped out like pus from a festering wound. I just nodded in response, sensing that her words and the feelings behind them needed no clarification, only acknowledgment.

Earlier that day, the nurse had informed me, Ms. Willis' life had sunk irreversibly into a pit. The doctor had given the bad news to her. I imagined his words, invading her mind like a poisonous gas: "Ma'am, you've tested HIV positive."

I moved my chair closer to Ms. Willis and offered her my hand. I wanted her to know that her diagnosis didn't scare me. I wanted her to know that it actually attracted me to her, for I suspected that if there was ever a time she needed to be touched, it was now. Despite her diagnosis, Ms. Willis was still in need of love and care. She was still human. In fact, she was closer to her humanity than she had ever been before.

Ms. Willis quickly grasped my hand, as if she didn't trust it would be there for very long. I wondered how many hands she would be denied in the years ahead. I wondered how many open arms she would be robbed of, and how many honest responses, intimate relationships, new opportunities would elude her. I wondered . . . How much love? How much life?

Suddenly Ms. Willis loosened her grip, letting her hand drop away. She looked up at me, taking a deep breath, as if this horrible news she had just received could be exhaled into oblivion. "Why don't they keep Bibles in the room?" she asked, seemingly pulling the question out of nowhere. I suspected that the reality of her new world was too much to handle now. After all, I was a chaplain and Bibles were easier to talk about.

"I can get you one if you like," I responded, attempting to skirt the irrelevant inquiry and address the motivation behind it.

"Yes, I'd like that," she replied. A sense of relief rushed over me with her request. Yes, a Bible was something I could provide. A cure for HIV infection? No way. A place of support and comfort? Questionable, but I was trying my best.

"You know the Unshackled Ministry in Chicago?" she asked, wearing a rare smile that exuded a few rays of hope and peace amid her darkness. "Well, I went there and it was so great. So many testimonies! You know . . . God really changes people's lives!"

"It sounds like that experience meant a lot to you," I echoed.

"Yes, it did," she responded. "I want to go there again . . . tomorrow!" Ms. Willis temporarily relaxed, resting her head on the pillow and looking up at the ceiling. Her thoughts appeared to be comforting her from the reality of her diagnosis that was surely cutting into her like a butcher knife.

"You could use some of that encouragement now, huh?" I offered, somewhat surprised that she hoped to make the trip so soon.

"Yeah, I sure could," she replied in a dreamlike voice. Apparently, Ms. Willis had already arrived at the Evangelical Christian ministry in her mind.

"Well, how about I go get that Bible now?" I blurted, unable to sustain the suffocating silence. Silence—a powerful presence that I seek to nurture in my ministry and in my life in general, only to repeatedly run away from it when it gets too close. I'm not sure I will ever learn to be totally comfortable with silence. It is foreign to my busy-bee, goal-oriented mind. It is foreign to the hospital in which I work, whose halls are filled with beeping machines, rushing doctors, and annoying overhead pages. Furthermore, it is foreign to

my culture, a people who seek to be stimulated by anything in order
to avoid thinking about what really matters.

"Would you like to have a prayer before I go?" I proposed,
making a desperate attempt to be helpful in some measurable way.
In the back of my mind, I knew that my offer was as much a plea to
ease my own discomfort as it was an extended hand to a woman
who had undoubtedly just received the worst news of her life.

"Dear Lord," I began. "Thank you for Ms. Willis, for the life
you have given her and for the person you have made her to be. We
pray that you would comfort her now . . ." It didn't take long before
my words were swallowed up by several loud sobs. Ms. Willis' face
collapsed into her chest, and the bed shook with each cry. Perhaps
she was realizing that the news of her diagnosis could not be ignored, that it had to be addressed, even if only with tears. Yes, Ms.
Willis was learning that while she could hide from the reality of her
HIV infection temporarily, but it never would go away completely.

As I sat next to Ms. Willis with my hand on her shoulder, words
and emotions began spouting from her lips like lava from an erupting volcano. "I'm just trying to think how I got this. I don't
know . . . I've been practicing safe sex for some time now. Was it
too late? I guess I did have a transfusion in seventy-nine. I don't do
drugs, like my sister. She's not going to believe this. And my son, I
tell him to wear a condom, but he don't. He don't listen to me. He
still can't get over the fact that I was in jail when he was a kid. I just
can't tell him about this. I don't know . . . And my other son, he's
just two. I bet he's wondering where Mama is. And my job. I'm a
cook. I hope my boss still lets me work . . ."

"It sounds like you have a lot of big questions on your mind, Ms.
Willis," I stated, reflecting the blatantly obvious. Her outpouring of
emotion left me feeling somewhat dumbfounded, not knowing
which of her concerns to address, if any at all. It was clear that Ms.
Willis had many issues to work through in the days and years ahead.

"It's understandable that you would have a lot of anxious questions," I continued. "You received some really difficult news to
hear." I wanted her to know that it was okay to cry, to get mad, to
have questions. I wanted her to know that it was okay to look at her
situation straight on and feel all the emotions that it provoked. In
fact, I suspected that this is what Ms. Willis needed to do in order to

move on to any sense of peace and hope. I thought of Shadrach, Meshach, and Abednigo, dancing in King Nebuchadnezzar's fiery furnace, as told in the book of Daniel (Daniel 3). Just as God *did not* promise to save the men from experiencing the fire, he *did not* promise to save Ms. Willis from contracting a life-threatening disease. But, just as he *did* promise to be with the men in the fire, he also *did* promise to be with Ms. Willis in her affliction.

Ms. Willis' tears continued to flow and her concerns continued to spill out. I just sat and listened, trying my best to provide a place where she could bring her grief, a place where she could share her burden for awhile. Eventually her emotional eruption subsided, as if she had run out of tears, worries, questions, as if she had run out of everything. Then I realized that Ms. Willis *had* run out of everything. She no longer had the control over her life that she thought she once had. I only hoped that she would realize in time that it was in losing her life that she would truly find it, that it was only in her emptiness that the God of all provision could fill her up.

31

Comfort in Death and in Life

My pager suddenly emitted its obnoxious beep at five-thirty that Easter morning, startling me from my restless slumber. In many ways, knowing a call could come at any moment was just as disconcerting as finally receiving it, as the anticipation had been holding me captive in a state of adrenaline-pumped vigilance all night long. It was my first weekend as the on-call chaplain; never before had I been given sole responsibility to minister to any of the patients in the hospital who might request a pastoral care visit. "Oh, Lord, please let it be a quiet weekend," I pleaded inside my head, imagining myself speechless amid a dying patient and weeping family members. And it *had* been relatively calm until that early Sunday morning, when I learned that God was inviting me to a new level of dependence and faithfulness. Yes, He called me forth from my hiding place in the call room, challenging me to be willing to go wherever He would lead me. As I headed to the pediatric emergency room, I took great comfort in the fact that I was not as alone as I thought I was.

"The baby stopped breathing, and Mrs. Abbot found him dead in the crib early this morning," Dr. Keller explained to me. I could hear the family in one of the adjacent examination rooms, mourning the loss of their four-month-old baby boy named Carl. Suddenly, Mrs. Abbot appeared in the doorframe of Room 3, looking as though she had been run over by a garbage truck. Her thick brown hair was matted down like a wet mop and her round face was splotchy, stained by the storm of tears that she was shedding. Dr. Keller introduced me to Mrs. Abbot, and immediately the grieving mother fell into my arms. As I held her long and tight, the weight of her body and the intensity of her immense sorrow permeated my entire being like a fast-acting yeast added to warm bread dough. "I can't believe this is happening!" she wailed. "It just doesn't make any sense."

Dr. Keller stood silently next to us with her arms crossed, looking down at the floor. She seemed not to know what to do, perhaps recognizing that there wasn't anything she could do. Certainly this uncomfortable realization was one that we both revisited time and time again in the hospital, sometimes courageous enough to use it to foster our humility, other times simply experiencing it as an assault to our pride. Wherever Dr. Keller was in that process, she finally spoke up as a sort of last resort. "The team did everything they could; they did a great job. But they just couldn't revive him." Her comment, while most likely well-meaning, seemed to serve like salt in an open wound, as Mrs. Abbot responded to it with a forceful sob. "Well, yeah, they obviously didn't do a good enough job!" I imagined this statement billowing inside her head, ushered by a wave of anger.

After a few minutes, Mrs. Abbot regained her stance, and we headed into the examination room where Baby Carl and the rest of his family were situated. Mr. Abbot stood in the far corner facing the wall, holding the lifeless body of his son. He cradled the little one in his arms, weeping over him and letting his tears drop on the baby's delicate cheeks. Swaddled in a cozy yellow blanket, Baby Carl looked as though he could simply be asleep, resting peacefully in his Father's care. In a sense, he was. In fact, if Baby Carl were to rise into the hands of God, that Easter morning seemed like an appropriate time to do so.

The site of Mr. Abbot embracing his beloved son left me speechless and motionless. I thought of God's reaching out to us when I saw the two of them, realizing that it is with the same painful passion that our Eternal Lover looks upon us, His broken children. Yes, just as Mr. Abbot's tears fell on the dear face of his Baby Carl, so do God's tears descend on our vulnerable hearts, cleansing us with His love to make way for whatever is to come. In this way, the father and son were a beautiful sight despite the agonizing circumstances. I stood in a holy awe for a moment, sensing that they both needed this poignant time together that could never be had again.

Mrs. Abbot and her other son, eight-year-old Marcus, sat in two of the cold and hard metal chairs that lined the wall, their loud cries echoing off the four bare walls. I pulled up another chair next to them, placing my hands on their shoulders in an attempt to caress a bit of comfort into their pain. Marcus planted his forehead into his hands, and mumbled the same words over and over again: "I just want to go home and go to sleep." I didn't know what to say in response, but then I realized that my acceptance of his feelings was all he needed at the time. "I know, I know . . ." I offered.

Marcus's and my attention shifted to Mrs. Abbot, whose head was bobbing up and down in a dire effort to enter some sort of rest. "My mother is trying to go to sleep so that she won't have to think about this," Marcus said. I sensed that the grieving boy was right; not only was he speaking of his mother, but also of himself. The only conceivable place for them to go at the moment was to the place of denial, to pretend it was all just a nightmare. Denial—the same mechanism that keeps us from healing also serves as its first step.

Suddenly, Baby Carl's grandmother and two cousins entered the room, bringing with them an additional surge of sorrow. Before I could introduce myself, I was embodied in a gigantic hug that included the entire family with Baby Carl in the middle. It didn't seem to matter that they knew who I was, only that they knew I was there with them. I felt more like a participant in the pain than a messenger of comfort, more like a part of the darkness than a proclaimer of the light. Ironically, I now realize that it was only through my being present in the pain and in the darkness that I was able to be of any comfort and light. In this way, I felt more like a sister than a chaplain. But then again, isn't that who I really am?

As we converged into a huddle, I thought of the scripture "For where two or three come together in my name, there am I with them" (Matthew 18:20). We were all members of God's team, not there to cheer on a victory, but rather to mourn a loss. And the loss was real, for it could not be repossessed, only remembered. It could not be cured, only remedied with the salve of faith and time. Not only did Baby Carl die that morning, but so also did the hopes and dreams he represented in the hearts of those who loved him. How honored I felt to be a part of that moment, for as we were bidding farewell to Baby Carl, we were also welcoming his tender and innocent spirit into our hearts. And in that process, we were also welcoming one another, and most important, God into our hearts. While Baby Carl's death appeared to be ripping everyone apart, in actuality, it was bringing broken hearts together to form a whole.

As we loosened our embrace, we all settled into a painful yet healing silence. Oddly enough, the Abbot family seemed to have found some of the comfort that they thought only Baby Carl could provide in one another. Yes, God *does* work in mysterious ways.

Toward the end of our time together, we all gathered for prayer, holding hands in a circle with Baby Carl on Mrs. Abbot's lap. "Dear Lord," I prayed, "we lift up Baby Carl and his loving family to you during this time of shock and sorrow . . ." My words were brief and to the point, as I sensed that somehow they had already been offered and already received. How comforting it was to know that in return, the God who received His people's pain also offered its only true remedy. The grief was far from over, but as a friend once told me, "Love and pain go together."

32

Home for the Holiday

The hallway of the cardiology floor was quieter than normal on that Thanksgiving Day. I imagined many of the nurses and doctors at home, welcoming aunts and uncles, stuffing turkeys, pinching the cheeks of the newest baby in the family, rooting for the underdog in the TV football game. The concerns here at the hospital were different, however. Mrs. Smith needed a new heart. Mr. Steinway couldn't be weaned from the ventilator. Mr. Bileray, known as one of many frequent flyers, had just landed his sixteenth visit of the year for chest pain. "Oh, him again!" I could see the nurses' faces exclaim.

Mrs. Franklin was different, however. The ninety-something African-American widow whose congestive heart failure kept her in and out of the hospital appeared as though her health was the least of her concerns. When I knocked on her door and introduced myself, Mrs. Franklin welcomed me like an honored guest. "Well, praise the Lord! Look who He has brought to me today!" I couldn't help but smile boldly in return, as her greeting made me feel special and wanted.

Many of the other patients' rooms were full of visitors, flowers, and cards, but Mrs. Franklin's space was bare and empty. This is what had led me to her room. "How sad and lonely she must be," I had thought to myself, wondering when her family would arrive for a holiday visit. Yet as I sat down at her bedside, the old woman exuded an inexhaustible peace that came from the warmth of her own spirit. In fact, her cheerful and appreciative demeanor brightened her room more than any floral arrangement or caring relative could. How strange it was to feel such intimate company in such a barren place.

Mrs. Franklin sat propped up in bed, her white hair perfectly braided into delicate strands that decorated her head. "Latisha did my hair! In'it beautiful?" I recall her exclaiming with a smile that showed as much gratitude as it did joy. Latisha was one of the nurse's aides; little did she know that on that Thanksgiving Day she was actually an angel wearing scrubs.

"I jis' lo-o-o-ve braids," Mrs. Franklin continued, in a spirit of reverie. "My mama used to do 'em when I was a youngin'. . . Mama, she was a good mama." She tilted her head to the side with a gentle smile, appearing to be temporarily suspended in a sort of nostalgia. The silence was quickly broken, however, when suddenly she was swept away into a flood of memories: Mama's corn pudding; the mean old neighbor on the farm who kicked the dog; Papa's drinking and the sounds of broken glass; the way her husband Raymond used to come up and pinch her in the behind while she did dishes at the kitchen sink; how he loved her even though she couldn't bear him any children . . . the words and images came and went, and with them the feelings and emotions they evoked. It occurred to me that I was being taken on a sacred journey without even leaving the room.

The time passed quickly but richly, and was brought to a close with the arrival of Thanksgiving dinner, a grand finale of sorts. With eyes the size of golf balls, Mrs. Franklin stared in anticipation at the turkey dinner tray in front of her, fresh from the hospital cafeteria. The same manufactured mashed potatoes and gravy-stained pumpkin pie that turned my stomach appeared to nourish hers even before she had a chance to take a bite. Ironically, the fragile woman looked more like a queen than a patient: the elevated bed served as her throne, the carefully constructed braids as her crown, and the dinner tray as her banquet table.

Mrs. Franklin's family never arrived that day. It occurred to me that the situation at her residence would have been no different. All the same, the little old woman's relatives were alive and well in her memory, and she appeared to be reliving both the joyful and painful moments with them as each story launched from her lips. What Mrs. Franklin's room lacked in visitors, it possessed in genuine company. What I had presumed would be her sadness had become her grounds for joy.

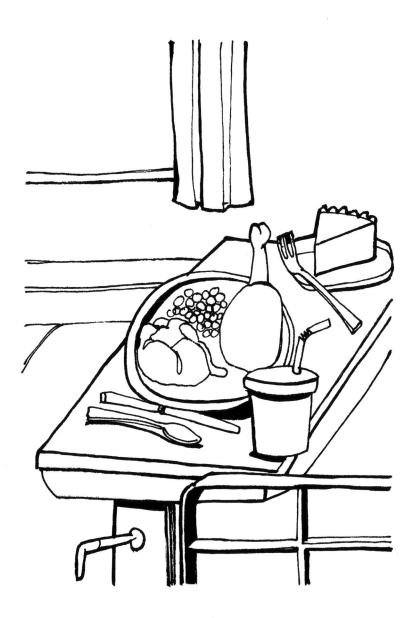

As I waved good-bye to Mrs. Franklin, I realized that here at the hospital she was actually as close to home as she could be. She not only had her memories to offer; but more important, she had an audience to receive them. She not only had laughter and tears; she had someone with whom to share them. She not only had a Thanksgiving feast; she had someone to prepare it for her. She not only had her delicate white hair; she had someone to braid it. She not only had life; she had a place to continue living, a place to give and receive, a place to love and be loved. Yes, it was a good time for Mrs. Franklin to be sick, for to have a place to call home may have been just the remedy her heart needed the most.

—33—

Everybody's Savior

Alisha and I had a lot in common, not in the degree of suffering we had both endured in our young lives, but rather in the similar issues that our suffering had evoked in our hearts and minds. In this way, ministering to Alisha was like ministering to myself. I was aware of this from the time of our first visit, knowing that our shared histories had the power to help or hinder my ability to provide pastoral care. Hoping to do the former, I asked God to enable me to put myself in her shoes, and to bring with me any of the wisdom and compassion He had revealed to me in my own trials.

Tapping on Alisha's door and hearing no response, I peered around the corner to find her in what I later learned was a drug-induced stupor. Apparently, the doctor had increased her dose of Demerol to help conquer the pain that her failing kidneys were causing. Before I could turn to leave Alisha in what I assumed was a rare escape from her chronic illness, the nurse's aide in the other side of the room aroused her from her slumber. "Alisha," she screeched. "You have a visitor!"

Alisha's limp body shook a few times, and then she tilted her head upright and blinked several times. I wished I could disappear from her blurry vision, fearing that the seventeen-year-old didn't want to be disturbed. It was my first day on that pediatric ward, and the last thing I wanted to do was cause an unnecessary flurry. But to my relief, Alisha's easy disposition immediately put me at ease.

"Oh, hi," she said, her soft voice touching me like a feather. After my brief introduction and apology, she invited me to have a seat at her bedside, treating me like an honored guest. She quickly pulled a comb through her hair and sprayed some Binaca in her mouth, and then arranged her purse, TV clicker, and pain pump control in a neat row on her sheets. I just watched, wondering for what she was so studiously preparing during our time together.

"So how are you feeling today?" I began.

"Well, I'm better than I was!" she proclaimed with a tired gasp. Her body seemed to sink into the bed like a sack of flour, mimicking the lethargy of her voice.

"It sounds like you've been through a lot," I reflected, hoping to call forth the story that I sensed she longed to tell.

"Oh, yeah . . . Ever since ninety-three, my life has been going downhill!" she agreed, her voice beginning to pick up momentum. "First I get kidney disease, and they don't even know what caused it. Then I get a transplant and sixteen other surgeries that don't work. And now, my family is falling apart. I just hate my life! I'm so tired of suffering!" She broke into sobs, not able to maintain the orderly façade she had initially tried so hard to project.

"It's okay to cry," I responded, stroking her sweat-stained hospital gown with my hand. Her lament permeated the room, each moan bouncing off the freshly sanitized tile floor. I wondered if she felt as alone as her surroundings looked, void of any cards and flowers, lacking a roommate or even a family member. Then I realized that after seventeen surgeries, the hospital was Alisha's second home, a place that *everyone* was tired of visiting, and Alisha herself, a person who perhaps had long ago worn out her reception into others' empathetic hearts. Alisha, the seemingly unsolvable problem, and the hospital, her convenient storage shelf.

Alisha's situation resonated with me, for amid four years of intractable bowel disease, I, too, hated my life and was tired of suffering. The gastroenterology clinic was my second home, and I, the doctors' "problem patient" and my family's relentless source of worry. I finally found physical relief after having my colon removed, and I now enjoy health. I only wished that Alisha's nightmare would have such a happy ending.

Alisha's outburst of emotion gave us many options for discussion: the surgeries, her family, what it was like to be in the hospital for the umpteenth time, the "why me" question, what her future would entail, hating life, and all of the feelings that these and other thoughts provoked. My heart ached with hers, knowing that the pain she must be feeling was similar to the hell that I had been through, only magnified and unique to her own experience. I sat there at a loss for words, not knowing which of her wounds needed the most immediate care, or if they could even be separated and prioritized at all. Deep down, however, I sensed that I needed only to acknowledge them in their totality and to accept Alisha in her brokenness, leaving any details to be shared up to her.

"I just found out that my mom is divorcing my dad," Alisha began, choosing the most recent catastrophe as a point of focus. "A couple of years ago, we was all fine. But now, Mom says she's gotta go." Alisha looked down into her lap, shaking her head in disbelief and disappointment.

"Mmmm," I responded, sensing a volcano of feelings on the verge of erupting. "How does that make you feel?"

"Angry!" she said vehemently. "My mom just isn't there! She lets my brother listen to any kind of rap music he wants, and I think we should just listen to gospel music. She even wants to pay my dad two thousand dollars for the divorce, but he won't take the money. I don't even know how she would pay him, she's used up all the credit cards! And now that I'm getting sicker, I can't do all the housework like I'm supposed to or look after my brothers."

"Yes, I can see why you'd be angry," I replied, affirming the feeling that she so readily admitted. As I listened to her, it occurred to me that Alisha wasn't experiencing her mother as a mother at all. In fact, it appeared that Alisha was assuming the role of a primary caregiver herself. I wondered if she had ever had a childhood, a time to be free to grow in the nurture and admonition of others, or if pain, suffering, and responsibilities were the only parts of life she knew.

Pain, suffering, and responsibilities. I once felt that these words solely characterized my life, too, only in a different way. Growing up with two sisters who seemed to push my parents' limits, I took on the role of the perfect child, feeling it was up to me to hold the family together. Straight "A's," a national tennis ranking, polite manners, and a slim body were the only answers; anything less was unacceptable. My life was not about exploration and discovery, as it is for most teens, but rather, about control and obligation. Perhaps Alisha was living by a similar set of rules.

"I just gotta do something!" she exclaimed, forming fists with her scaly and swollen hands. "My brothers need a mother to grow up with, especially when I'm no longer around. I just gotta do something!" I just listened, noting in the back of my mind that Alisha had already so bravely acknowledged the fact that her life was not in her own hands. I wondered when she would realize that her family's life was not, either.

"Maybe there isn't anything you can do," I replied, feeling as though I was going out on a limb, not knowing if she was ready to hear such a painful reality. At the same time, I knew that this truth could be freeing for her, as it was for me. I'll never forget the strange sense of relief I felt after losing a tennis match to someone ranked several spots behind me, and then discovering that everyone, including myself, was still okay. "You mean life just goes on?" I remember thinking to myself amid the shame and embarrassment the event had provoked inside me. "You mean others will still accept me, my coach will still work with me, and my parents won't be disappointed in me?" How liberating it was to realize that the world didn't revolve around me as I thought it had.

"But if I don't do something, nobody else will," Alisha pleaded, trying her best to hold onto the notion that everybody needed her to be their savior. Strangely, the same identity that was sucking all of the life out of her was the same one that she clung to for a sense of purpose. Her imploring response echoed loudly in my memory, calling forth all of the times I have said the same thing. "But if I don't go to see Grandmère at the nursing home, no one else will." Or "But if I don't take out the trash, no one else will." Even though no one ever asked me for my assistance, I assumed that their affairs were my responsibility, that they would be ruined without my immediate attendance. Yes, Alisha and I shared codependency in common: our giving personalities could mutate into destructive coping mechanisms, our attributes becoming our own worst enemies.

"Hmm, that's an awful lot of responsibility for a young person to bear," I reflected, hoping she would come to see the impossible position in which she was placing herself. Alisha had a choice to make: she could continue to try to give out of the poverty of her own self, or she could seek God to give out of the abundance of His blessings within her. Little did she know that the God who dwelt within her was all that she and everyone else needed.

Alisha and I met several times after our first visit, sometimes talking more about her struggles, sometimes nurturing a rare moment of silence, and sometimes just watching TV together. Other times we would take field trips to the rec room to play pool. Often Alisha barely had the strength to hold the pool stick, looking as though she might collapse right onto the green felt table. But her determination kept her going, in more ways than one. "I'll be okay," she would always say in response to my continual expressions of concern. "I'm used to this." Yes, Alisha was accustomed to suffering, a constant state that seemed to both nurture and destroy her hope for whatever was to come.

I often check the hospital census to see if Alisha is back in the hospital, perhaps for her eighteenth surgery. I look for her name with both longing and foreboding, for while her pain is severe and her problems unsolvable, her genuine emotions that emanate from them strike a chord in my heart. I have traveled through the same desolate abyss of chronic illness, and I know what it feels like to try to be everybody's sacrificial lamb. In Alisha, I found a home for my own hurts, a secure place where I know that I am not alone. In her weakness, I found comfort. "Please come back if I'm here again, Gretchen," she requested at her time of discharge. I was honored to know that she had found the same safe place in me.

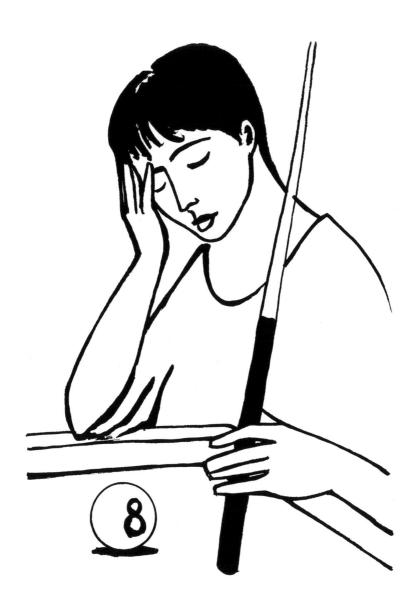

34

And God Was in It All

Mr. Carson sat stiff and upright in his bedside chair. He appeared on the verge of tears, his lower lip quivering over his upper lip, as if to keep it sealed shut. His eyes shimmered with escaped tears, staring down at his blood-stained hospital gown. I had just come in to introduce myself, to let him know that chaplains were available, yet I could tell I was walking into a tense time for this fifty-something man whose rough looks couldn't mask his fear, as hard as he tried.

"They keep putting it off!" he finally blurted out.

"Hmm . . . they keep putting it off," I reflected back to him. I had no idea what he was talking about—an impending surgery, his discharge, a meal change from clear to full liquid—but somehow I knew that it really didn't matter whether I knew. What mattered was the feeling with which Mr. Carson made his statement. He was frustrated, and he needed his feelings to be acknowledged. "That sounds really frustrating," I said, trying my best to be what he needed at that moment. "This must be a hard time for you."

Mr. Carson burst into tears. It was like watching a dam burst. I kneeled beside him with my hand on his shoulder. I just sat with him in the midst of his misery. "It's okay," I said softly. Behind my words were feelings of temptation to break in and say, "Oh, don't cry!" But I knew that was my own insecurity at work, not the spirit of God in me. So, I resisted the temptation and stayed in the moment. Mr. Carson was overflowing with fear, hurt, and anger, and this is where he needed to be. And that is where God was, too. So that is where I wanted to be. "Ahh," I thought to myself, "now the healing can begin."

But suddenly, Mr. Carson's tidal wave of tears dried up, his stiff upper lip reformed and his eyes refocused on his gown. He appeared as if he felt ashamed. "I'll be okay, lady," he uttered under his breath.

"Oh, brother," I thought to myself. "What did I do?" Mr. Carson seemed to turn off from me. Did I push him too hard? Did I make him feel threatened? Or, was it just a scary place for him to be? Did he simply feel too vulnerable to cry in front of a stranger, to cry at all? Did he feel the need to "pull himself up by his bootstraps" in order to cope with the situation? All of these possibilities raced through my mind as we sat in silence. No matter what happened, I couldn't help but feel like a failure in some respects.

Failure. The word is one that floats through my mind regularly as a chaplain. It looms inside my head as I try to figure out what went awry, and then it descends to the pit of my stomach, leaving me with an empty feeling. It is easy to take patients' reactions personally, to look back and wish I *hadn't* done this or said that, or to wish that I *had* done this or said that. "Hindsight is twenty-twenty," one of my supervisors used to say.

But whatever happened with Mr. Carson, whatever allowed him to open up and whatever caused him to close up, however I helped him or hindered him, my faith tells me that God was in it all. It was the God of compassion in me that brought Mr. Carson to a safe place where he could cry and share his frustration. It was the God of infinite grace in Mr. Carson who allowed him to reclaim a sort of denial, a place where he needed to be at that time. And now, it is the God of humility in me who enables me to evaluate my own response to Mr. Carson's words and actions.

As I move on from my experience with Mr. Carson, my faith continues to tell me that God is in all that lies ahead. God goes with me, for it is the God of renewal in me who enables me to be pruned and to grow from what I learn about others, myself, and life in general. And finally, it is the God of faithfulness in me who strengthens me to return to those who hurt, even when I feel incapable of helping and unable to offer any peaceful presence.

35

Pink Pajamas in Heaven

Mrs. Walker's room was empty. A flicker of excitement rushed through my mind as I stood motionless in the hallway, staring at the freshly starched linens and shiny linoleum floors that now reclaimed her space.

"She got a heart . . . she got a heart . . ." I said to myself slowly. I felt paralyzed, trapped among feelings of shock, elation, and dread, intensely curious yet afraid to know more. I had been waiting for this day for several months, and needless to say, so had Mrs. Walker.

Several nurses brushed past me busily, from bedside to medication cart to ECG monitor to patient chart. It quickly became apparent to me that the Cardiac Care Unit didn't have time for my daze.

"Excuse me," I uttered to one of the nurses on her way to the break room.

"Yeah?" she responded in a cheerful manner not often seen in a profession that demands more than can be given.

"Mrs. Walker . . . do you know if she got her heart?" My question seemed to hang in the air for an eternity.

"Yes, she did."

I sighed with relief, closing my eyes and tilting my head backward. "Oh, wonderful!" I replied, already envisioning myself rushing over to the Cardiac Surgical Intensive Care Unit to check on her postoperative condition.

"But she rejected it. She died." The nurse's words dug into me like a sledgehammer. I felt as if my heart had been thrown into an abyss, only to hit the bottom and crack.

"She died?" I queried, as if uncertain that what I was experiencing was real. Mrs. Walker wasn't the type to just die. She was a survivor, a fighter. "I have too much to live for," she once said to me, pointing to a picture of her eight-year-old daughter whose drawings covered the walls.

"Yeah, we were all really surprised. I had just talked to her the day before she went to the OR," the nurse recounted. "It's so sad," she continued, shaking her head, then fetching her lunch from the beeping microwave. Apparently, the CCU didn't have time for anything still or silent, even death.

The break room no longer felt like a refuge from the busy hallways; it took on a repulsive character. I sat in one of the cold, hard chairs, resting my head in my arms on the table and staring blankly at the mustard packets and want ads that littered its surface. Everything around me seemed temporarily meaningless, void of any value or worth.

"Why did you let this happen?!" I yelled inside my head to God. I felt angry, cheated from justice, robbed of the hope that I had had, of the hope that Mrs. Walker had had. "Why does it seem the good ones always die, Lord?" The "why" questions circled my mind like a swarm of buzzing bees.

It just didn't make sense. Mrs. Walker was too kind, too courageous, too strong, too alive for death. The forty-one-year-old woman who had suffered from a cardiomyopathy most of her life occupied a special place in my heart. We had enjoyed several lengthy conversations together in that room in which she had been held captive for six months. We talked about everything from the waiting for her heart, to her husband and daughter she loved, to the endless trays of bland hospital food, to Saint Teresa to whom she prayed, and then back to the waiting. Yes, the waiting: this seemed to be the only constant in her life, and even it, too, was uncertain. "The waiting is hard," she said one time. "And sometimes I just need to cry because I get so discouraged. But I know I need to be strong through this. I just know I will get through this." We never talked about death. It never seemed to be an option.

Mrs. Walker was much more than an optimist. She seemed to be able to feel and acknowledge the painful gravity of her situation, yet she also seemed to be able to rise above it. "I have my own pity party from time to time," she once admitted to me, with the gentle smile that so often graced her face. "But God is still good. He's still in this." I remember being amazed with her courageous outlook, envisioning myself sobbing in a desperate heap if I were in such a situation. She was one of the few patients I have ever met who was able to live her predicament to the fullest, neither stuck in the bowels of despair nor riding the relentless wave of denial. Mrs. Walker seemed to maintain a healthy medium. If only her body had been as strong as her spirit.

I take Mrs. Walker with me in a visible way as I visit other patients in the hospital. Her quirky question, posed one day with a big smile, pinched nose, and tilted head, remains fixed in my memory. "May I ask you a question?" she said out of the blue.

"Sure," I responded, wondering what I was getting myself into.

"Why do chaplains always wear such dark and boring colors?" She pointed toward the khaki pants and sweater I had thoughtlessly pulled from my closet that morning. "You should wear something happier. It's already too dark and dreary being in here."

I reflected briefly on her straightforward comment, noticing that Mrs. Walker herself was adorned in pink silk pajamas most likely brought from home. It was striking to me how much more hope she exuded in this attire as opposed to the ratty, gray hospital gowns that most patients wore. "You know," I responded, still somewhat captured by the insight and practicality of her observation, "that's a great idea. I'm going to think of you every time I get dressed in the morning!" We both laughed, and everything around us seemed to take on a brighter hue.

Looking back to the morning when I learned of Mrs. Walker's death, it is no wonder that I had chosen a cheery, light blue, floral dress to wear that day. It seemed only natural as I was standing in my daze, staring into her empty room. Even though she was no longer sitting restlessly on her bed in her pink pajamas, casting her smile that seemed to brighten the entire CCU, I could still hear her speaking to me in a joyful tone. "Oh, I love that dress, Gretchen. It's so happy!" I wonder if Mrs. Walker is wearing her pink pajamas in heaven.

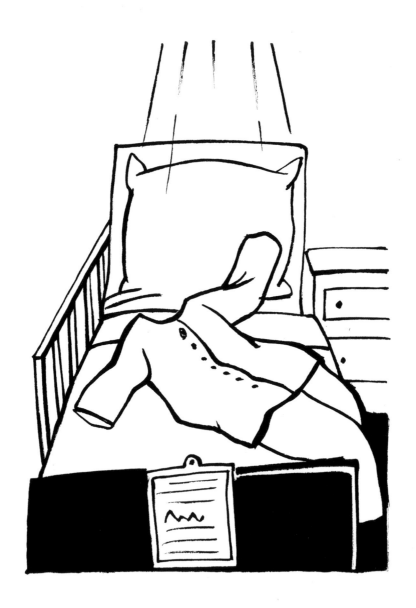

©1999 Michael O'Neill McGrath, OSFS

Order Your Own Copy of
This Important Book for Your Personal Library!

BROKEN BODIES, HEALING HEARTS
Reflections of a Hospital Chaplain

_____ in hardbound at $49.95 (ISBN: 0-7890-0851-3)

_____ in softbound at $19.95 (ISBN: 0-7890-0852-1)

COST OF BOOKS_____

OUTSIDE USA/CANADA/
MEXICO: ADD 20%_____

POSTAGE & HANDLING_____
(US: $3.00 for first book & $1.25
for each additional book)
Outside US: $4.75 for first book
& $1.75 for each additional book)

SUBTOTAL_____

IN CANADA: ADD 7% GST_____

STATE TAX_____
(NY, OH & MN residents, please
add appropriate local sales tax)

FINAL TOTAL_____
(If paying in Canadian funds,
convert using the current
exchange rate. UNESCO
coupons welcome.)

☐ **BILL ME LATER:** ($5 service charge will be added)
(Bill-me option is good on US/Canada/Mexico orders only;
not good to jobbers, wholesalers, or subscription agencies.)

☐ Check here if billing address is different from
shipping address and attach purchase order and
billing address information.

Signature_____

☐ **PAYMENT ENCLOSED: $**_____

☐ **PLEASE CHARGE TO MY CREDIT CARD.**

☐ Visa   ☐ MasterCard   ☐ AmEx   ☐ Discover
☐ Diners Club
Account #_____

Exp. Date_____

Signature_____

Prices in US dollars and subject to change without notice.

NAME _____

INSTITUTION _____

ADDRESS _____

CITY _____

STATE/ZIP _____

COUNTRY _____ COUNTY (NY residents only) _____

TEL _____ FAX _____

E-MAIL_____
May we use your e-mail address for confirmations and other types of information? ☐ Yes   ☐ No

Order From Your Local Bookstore or Directly From
The Haworth Press, Inc.
10 Alice Street, Binghamton, New York 13904-1580 • USA
TELEPHONE: 1-800-HAWORTH (1-800-429-6784) / Outside US/Canada: (607) 722-5857
FAX: 1-800-895-0582 / Outside US/Canada: (607) 772-6362
E-mail: getinfo@haworthpressinc.com
PLEASE PHOTOCOPY THIS FORM FOR YOUR PERSONAL USE.

BOF96